WHY ME?

THE BRAIN ON TILT

WHY ME?

THE BRAIN ON TILT

by

David A. Kent, M.D. Psychiatrist

Why Me? : The Brain on Tilt
David A. Kent, M.D. Psychiatrist

Paperback Edition ISBN: 979-8-9937794-0-9
Hardcover Edition ISBN: 979-8-9937794-2-3

Flames Creations | Design Services Provided by Flames Creations

CONTENTS

WHY ME? THE BRAIN ON TILT

AUTHOR'S INTRODUCTION

When I decided to write this book, I didn't do it from the comfortable distance of clinical detachment. I did it from a place of necessity—the necessity that comes from watching people you love struggle with conditions that are profoundly misunderstood, deeply stigmatized, and often treatable if only people knew the truth about them.

Over the past thirty-four years of psychiatric practice—since 1990—I have had the privilege of working with thousands of individuals battling mental illness. I have seen the transformative power of medication management, the remarkable recovery possible with evidence-based psychotherapy, and the life-changing potential of advanced interventions like transcranial magnetic stimulation (TMS) and electroconvulsive therapy (ECT). I have witnessed people reclaim their lives, rebuild their relationships, and rediscover their potential.

But I have also witnessed something far more painful: I have watched brilliant, talented, resilient people—including several of my own children—struggle not only with mental illness itself, but with the crushing weight of shame, isolation, and stigma that surrounds it. I have seen capable individuals avoid treatment because they feared being labeled "crazy" or "broken." I have watched families suffer in silence, unsure how to help or afraid of being judged for having mental illness "run in the family."

These personal experiences transformed my understanding of my work. I realized that my role as a psychiatrist extended beyond prescribing medications and managing symptoms—it extended to changing hearts and minds. It meant helping the world understand that mental illness is not a character flaw, a sign of weakness, or a moral failing. Mental illness is medicine. It is biology. It is brain chemistry, neural circuits, and neurotransmitter dysfunction that responds to treatment just as diabetes responds to insulin or hypertension responds to antihypertensive medication.

This book is my attempt to do that work of transformation.

THE MISSION: SCIENCE AND STORY

Throughout my career, I have been shaped by extraordinary mentors whose contributions to psychiatry have fundamentally altered how we understand and treat mental illness.

Dr. Donald W. Black, an exceptionally prolific clinical researcher with over 400 peer-reviewed publications, taught me the rigorous discipline of evidence-based practice. Dr. George Winokur, whose seminal work on diagnostic criteria and the genetics of mood disorders laid the foundation for modern psychiatric classification, showed me how rigorous science could bring clarity to seemingly chaotic conditions. Dr. William Coryell, Professor Emeritus at the University of Iowa Carver College of Medicine and author of over 375 publications, demonstrated how long-term longitudinal research could illuminate the natural history of mental illness and guide treatment decisions. And Dr. Nancy Andreasen—a visionary who received the National Medal of Science from President Clinton for her pivotal contributions to understanding the integration of mind, brain, and behavior through neuroimaging—showed me that breakthrough understanding comes from courageously applying new technologies and asking bold questions about the nature of consciousness and mental illness.

From these mentors, I learned that scientific rigor is essential—but I also learned, through three decades of practice, that science alone is incomplete. Numbers, statistics, and neurotransmitter systems tell us how mental illness works, but stories tell us why it matters. Stories remind us that behind every diagnosis is a human being—someone's daughter or son, someone's parent or partner, someone with dreams and potential and capacity for recovery.

This book bridges that gap. It combines rigorous science with compelling human narratives. It presents the biological foundations of mental illness—the brain structures, neurotransmitter systems, and neuroplasticity that underpin both illness and recovery. It addresses the myths and misconceptions that fuel stigma. And it tells the stories of real people (with names and identifying details changed to protect privacy) whose lives have been transformed by proper diagnosis and evidence-based treatment.

HOW THIS BOOK IS ORGANIZED

Part I: Foundation (Chapters 1-3) establishes the scientific and conceptual bedrock for everything that follows. Chapter 1 explores the remarkable complexity of the human brain and explains why mental illness is fundamentally a medical issue, not a moral one. Chapter 2 directly confronts the seven most damaging myths about mental illness, using data and research to reveal the truth beneath these misconceptions. Chapter 3 explores personality types and personality disorders, showing how personality intersects with mental illness and how guided therapeutic decisions offer hope for meaningful change.

Part II: Stories from the Mind (Chapters 4-9) presents six detailed case studies of individuals navigating different mental illnesses. We follow a high-functioning marketing manager through major depression and recovery. We journey with Marcus, a brilliant software engineer whose manic episode leads to bipolar disorder diagnosis and remarkable stability through treatment. We meet an engineering student whose schizophrenia onset derailed his dreams of becoming an engineer and how he navigated his life thereafter. We encounter individuals with obsessive-compulsive disorder, borderline personality disorder, and schizoaffective disorder—conditions often misunderstood but highly treatable. Through these stories, we see how mental illness affects real people, how diagnosis brings clarity, and how proper treatment enables recovery and fulfillment.

Part III: Hope, Treatment, and Moving Forward (Chapters 10-12) focuses on solutions. Chapter 9 explores the science of treatment—the evidence-based therapies and medications that work, including advanced approaches like ketamine therapy, TMS, and ECT. Chapter 10 examines the critical role of family and support systems in recovery, with practical strategies for communication, crisis management, and healing. Chapter 11 offers a message of hope grounded in three decades of clinical experience: recovery is possible, lives can be rebuilt, and mental illness, while serious, is manageable with proper treatment and support.

WHY THIS BOOK MATTERS NOW

We live in a time of unprecedented mental health crisis. Rates of depression, anxiety, and suicide have climbed steadily over the past two decades. Young people report more mental health struggles than any previous generation. Stigma, however, remains stubbornly resistant—many people still believe that having mental illness means being fundamentally broken or dangerous, that seeking treatment is a sign of weakness, or that recovery is unlikely.

Nothing could be further from the truth.

The evidence is overwhelming: mental illness is treatable. The human brain is remarkably plastic and capable of recovery. With proper diagnosis, evidence-based medication management, effective psychotherapy, lifestyle modifications, and strong support systems, individuals with mental illness can achieve not just symptom management but genuine flourishing. They can work meaningful jobs, maintain loving relationships, pursue their passions, and contribute to their communities.

But this recovery depends, first, on understanding. It depends on people recognizing that mental illness is real, medical, and treatable. It depends on families understanding how to support their loved ones rather than shame them. It depends on individuals recognizing that seeking help is an act of courage and wisdom, not weakness.

This book is my contribution to that essential work of understanding. It is written for anyone touched by mental illness—whether you live with it yourself, love someone who does, work in mental health, or simply want to understand the human mind better. It is written with the conviction that knowledge reduces stigma, that stories humanize statistics, and that hope, grounded in evidence and experience, has genuine power to transform lives.

A PERSONAL NOTE

This book is dedicated to everyone who struggles with mental illness, and especially to my own family members who have faced these battles with remarkable courage and resilience. Your struggles made me a better clinician. Your recovery gave me hope. Your willingness to be honest about mental health challenges—even within our own family—taught me that destigmatization begins at home.

My own research journey has reinforced this commitment. My early work on conversion disorders (1987-1995) contributed to our understanding of functional neurological disorders and remains cited in contemporary medical literature and DSM criteria. More recently, my post marketing data on FDA-approved Deep TMS technology and post-marketing surveillance studies has advanced our understanding of neurostimulation's durability and treatment response predictors. This work—spanning foundational research to clinical translation—has convinced me that rigorous science, combined with compassionate practice, can genuinely transform lives.

To my mentors—Drs. Black, Winokur, Coryell, and Andreasen—thank you for showing me what rigorous science looks like, what intellectual courage means, and how psychiatry can change lives. Your legacy is present on every page of this book.

To my patients over the past thirty-four years: thank you for trusting me with your most vulnerable moments, for teaching me through your struggles and your recoveries, and for showing me that mental illness, while serious, never defines the totality of a human being.

And to my readers: I invite you into this exploration of the mind with an open heart. If you are struggling with mental illness, I want you to know that you are not alone, you are not broken, and recovery is possible. If you love someone struggling, know that understanding and compassion matter profoundly. If you work in mental health, I hope this book affirms the vital importance of your work. And if you are simply curious about the human mind, I believe you will find both science and wisdom in these pages.

The mind is our most complex organ. But it is not unknowable. And mental illness, while challenging, is not insurmountable.

Let's begin the journey of understanding.

ABOUT THE AUTHOR

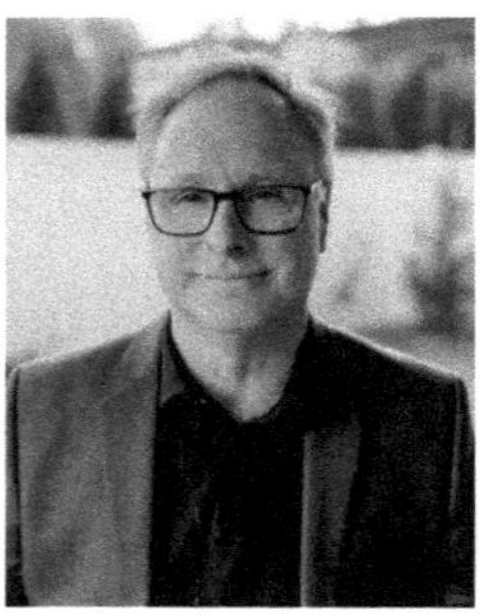

David Kent, M.D. is a board-certified psychiatrist with over three decades of clinical experience in medication management, inpatient and outpatient psychiatric care, and advanced brain stimulation techniques including transcranial magnetic stimulation (TMS) and electroconvulsive therapy (ECT). In private practice since 1990, he has worked with thousands of individuals across the full spectrum of mental illness, witnessing both the profound challenges these conditions present and the remarkable potential for recovery with proper treatment. His clinical work has been informed by mentorship under some of psychiatry's most influential figures, and his personal commitment to destigmatizing mental illness drives his ongoing work as a clinician, educator, and advocate.

PART I

FOUNDATION

CHAPTER 1
THE HUMAN BRAIN – OUR MOST COMPLEX ORGAN

The human brain weighs three pounds and contains 86 billion neurons, each connected to thousands of others through a maze of networks.[1] The internet pales in comparison. The brain consumes 20% of our body's energy, despite being approximately 2% of total body weight.[2] This relatively small organ produces consciousness, emotions, memory, and everything we experience and are capable of doing.

For whatever reason, we apply different standards to the brain than to other organs such as the heart. In fact, when I was in medical school, a cardiologist who found out I was going into psychiatry remarked that I would be leaving the practice of medicine. Such was the attitude I had to face going into the field. While we accept that other organs can fail—the heart with arrhythmias, kidneys with renal failure, the pancreas with dysfunction leading to diabetes—we struggle to understand that brains can develop depression, psychosis, and anxiety. This disconnect contributes to the stigma surrounding mental illness, preventing people and families from seeking help.

THE BIOLOGY OF MENTAL ILLNESS

The biology of mental illness is an ongoing area of intense research worldwide. It involves studying the complex relationship between genetics, brain structure and function, and neurochemistry.

Schizophrenia, bipolar disorder, and major depressive disorder are highly heritable, meaning that some individuals are genetically predisposed.[3] Environmental factors also play a role, interacting with these genetic factors. These include stress, trauma, infection, and substance use. All of these factors, combined with genetic predisposition, can alter brain development and function. That is why we often don't see illnesses like schizophrenia or bipolar disorder fully emerge until the late teens or early twenties—the brain doesn't fully mature until then.[4]

The biological basis of mental illness comes from many areas of research. Brain imaging studies show structural and functional differences in conditions like schizophrenia, bipolar disorder, and major depressive disorder.[5]

My first exposure to this was in 1985 when I was a research assistant for Dr. Nancy Andreason, MD, at the University of Iowa Hospitals and Clinics as a senior (4th year) medical student. She was a pioneer in schizophrenia research and was one of the first to use MRI imaging of schizophrenic brains. I remember tracing actual schizophrenic brain images onto paper to measure any size differences between those brains and normal controls. Although it seemed pretty rudimentary at the time, it was exciting to be at the forefront of that research, working with a world-renowned psychiatrist and author. She later received the National Medal of Science—America's highest award for scientific achievement—from President Clinton in 2000 for her pivotal contributions.[6] Over time, advanced brain imaging has revealed reduced gray matter volume in specific regions and disrupted networks in schizophrenia.[7]

Bipolar disorder is one of the most heritable psychiatric illnesses, with twin studies estimating heritability at 70-80%.[8] Bipolar disorder is associated with dysregulation of key neurotransmitters including dopamine, serotonin, and norepinephrine, which are central to mood, reward, and arousal.[9] The effectiveness of mood stabilizer medications that target these neurotransmitters further supports this connection. Inflammation has also been implicated in individuals with bipolar disorder, with increased markers of inflammation pointing to a potential role.[10]

The limbic system in the brain plays a key role in various mental illnesses. It's the emotional "engine" in the brain as well as the center for storing memory. It is also connected to the prefrontal cortex, which is part of a circuit referred to as the prefrontal-limbic-striatal network.[11] TMS (transcranial magnetic stimulation) works through these types of networks, directly stimulating key areas of the limbic system. The limbic system is very old from an evolutionary standpoint and is found in all mammals. We share the same range and types of emotions, creating a biological kinship. Depression, anxiety, and likely PTSD (post-traumatic stress disorder) have links to the limbic system.[12]

Key components of the limbic system include:

The amygdala processes fear, anxiety, pleasure, emotional memories, and triggers the "fight or flight" response.[13]

The hippocampus forms new long-term memories, is involved in learning, and regulates the stress hormone cortisol. It may actually shrink during prolonged depressive episodes.[14]

The hypothalamus regulates the stress response, sleep, appetite, and sex drive. This region has been implicated in depression and bipolar disorder.[15]

The nucleus accumbens is the reward center for motivation, pleasure, and reinforcement learning. Addiction can be linked to this region.[16]

The anterior cingulate cortex (ACC) integrates emotion and motivation and is key to error detection and emotional regulation. OCD (obsessive-compulsive disorder), schizophrenia, and depression have been associated with this region as well.[17]

The prefrontal cortex (PFC), or the "brain's brakes," generally regulates the limbic system.[18]

Suffice it to say, the limbic system and its connections to other brain regions are critical to our understanding of mental illness.

Understanding how the various regions of the brain function and interact with each other is critical to understanding the complex nature of the brain. The brain is like the last frontier of medical research. It is considered one of the most complex "machines" in the universe. Although the latest supercomputers and AI are advancing at incredible speed, no supercomputer has been able to outpace the brain in energy efficiency, adaptive learning, contextual understanding, and managing whole-body systems with minimal power consumption.[19] There is no doubt that with brute force, AI will catch up and surpass humans in many areas, but not as efficiently. Consider that the brain weighs only three pounds and what it can accomplish.

This is what makes mental illness particularly difficult to fully understand from a biological standpoint. In contrast to a broken bone, which is pretty straightforward, a "broken brain" is far more complex and interconnected. A person with bipolar disorder doesn't just experience mood swings but also struggles with impaired judgment during manic or depressive episodes, disrupted sleep patterns, altered energy levels, and challenges maintaining relationships and employment. This complexity is why mental health treatment usually requires a multifaceted approach. Medications play a critical role, but lifestyle interventions like exercise, sleep hygiene, and stress management cannot be overlooked.[20] Family support also plays a crucial role.

THE ROLE OF PERSONALITY

Psychiatrists tend to view personality disorders as pervasive, enduring, and inflexible patterns of thinking and feeling—behaviors that significantly deviate from cultural expectations, causing substantial distress and functional impairment.[21] The role of biology in personality is supported by a heritability rate of around 50%.[22] However, environmental factors play in considerably, such as early childhood trauma, neglect, abuse, and chronic stress leading to maladaptive patterns. Neurotransmitter abnormalities and problems in brain circuits regulating emotion and impulse control have been implicated in many personality disorders.[23]

One central issue with individuals with personality disorders is egosyntonicity, meaning they often don't see their personality traits as the problem but rather see other people or the world as flawed. Personality disorders can co-occur with other mental illnesses, making them more challenging to treat. Personality disorders typically require longer-term psychotherapy focused on ingrained patterns of thinking and behaving. This relies on the individual recognizing the need for treatment in the first place.

THE IMPORTANCE OF EARLY RECOGNITION

Unrecognized and untreated mental illness leads to poor outcomes. The average delay between the onset of symptoms and treatment ranges between 6-20 years.[24] This delay leads to deterioration of relationships, careers, and housing, and has secondary effects like increased substance use disorders, criminal behavior, and incarceration.[25]

Early recognition and intervention dramatically improve outcomes. Early intervention seems to improve response rates to medications, therapy, and other biological interventions such as TMS (transcranial magnetic stimulation).[26] By addressing personality disorders in young adults, we can prevent decades of interpersonal chaos and self-destructive behaviors.

Parents, teachers, friends, and colleagues are critical to being the first to notice someone struggling and encourage early intervention. I'm always relieved when I see a patient who has insight. They will likely engage in treatment and be more compliant, with far better outcomes. Those without insight need others to encourage them to stay in treatment; otherwise, the outcome will be poor.

MOVING FORWARD

As we explore specific mental health conditions and personality types in the coming chapters, remember this fundamental truth: mental illness is not a choice, a weakness, or a character flaw. Rather, it's a medical condition affecting the body's most complex organ. I will share stories of people that are examples of common mental health conditions that may ring true to examples you have come across. The central message is that mental illness is common, treatable, and nothing to be ashamed of. This is important because we are all touched by mental illness, either directly or indirectly.

FOOTNOTES

1. Herculano-Houzel, S. (2009). The human brain in numbers: a linearly scaled-up primate brain. *Frontiers in Human Neuroscience, 3*, 31.

2. Raichle, M. E., & Gusnard, D. A. (2002). Appraising the brain's energy budget. *Proceedings of the National Academy of Sciences, 99*(16), 10237-10239.

3. Sullivan, P. F., Kendler, K. S., & Neale, M. C. (2003). Schizophrenia as a complex trait: evidence from a meta-analysis of twin studies. *Archives of General Psychiatry, 60*(12), 1187-1192.

4. Gogtay, N., Giedd, J. N., Lusk, L., et al. (2004). Dynamic mapping of human cortical development during childhood through early adulthood. *Proceedings of the National Academy of Sciences, 101*(21), 8174-8179.

5. Goodkind, M., Eickhoff, S. B., Oathes, D. J., et al. (2015). Identification of a common neurobiological substrate for mental illness. *JAMA Psychiatry, 72*(4), 305-315.

6. National Science Foundation. (2000). The President's National Medal of Science: Recipient Details - Nancy C. Andreasen. Retrieved from https://www.nsf.gov/od/nms/recip_details.jsp?recip_id=10

7. van Erp, T. G., Hibar, D. P., Rasmussen, J. M., et al. (2016). Subcortical brain volume abnormalities in 2028 individuals with schizophrenia and 2540 healthy controls via the ENIGMA consortium. *Molecular Psychiatry, 21*(4), 547-553.

8. McGuffin, P., Rijsdijk, F., Andrew, M., Sham, P., Katz, R., & Cardno, A. (2003). The heritability of bipolar affective disorder and the genetic relationship to unipolar depression. *Archives of General Psychiatry, 60*(5), 497-502.

9. Cousins, D. A., Butts, K., & Young, A. H. (2009). The role of dopamine in bipolar disorder. *Bipolar Disorders, 11*(8), 787-806.

10. Goldstein, B. I., Kemp, D. E., Soczynska, J. K., & McIntyre, R. S. (2009). Inflammation and the phenomenology, pathophysiology, comorbidity, and treatment of bipolar disorder: a systematic review of the literature. *Journal of Clinical Psychiatry, 70*(8), 1078-1090.

11. Price, J. L., & Drevets, W. C. (2010). Neurocircuitry of mood disorders. *Neuropsychopharmacology, 35*(1), 192-216.

12. Rauch, S. L., Shin, L. M., & Phelps, E. A. (2006). Neurocircuitry models of posttraumatic stress disorder and extinction: human neuroimaging research—past, present, and future. *Biological Psychiatry, 60*(4), 376-382.

13. LeDoux, J. E. (2000). Emotion circuits in the brain. *Annual Review of Neuroscience, 23*(1), 155-184.

14. Sheline, Y. I., Gado, M. H., & Kraemer, H. C. (2003). Untreated depression and hippocampal volume loss. *American Journal of Psychiatry, 160*(8), 1516-1518.

15. Nemeroff, C. B., & Vale, W. W. (2005). The neurobiology of depression: inroads to treatment and new drug discovery. *Journal of Clinical Psychiatry, 66*(Suppl 7), 5-13.

16. Nestler, E. J., & Carlezon, W. A. (2006). The mesolimbic dopamine reward circuit in depression. *Biological Psychiatry, 59*(12), 1151-1159.

17. Bush, G., Luu, P., & Posner, M. I. (2000). Cognitive and emotional influences in anterior cingulate cortex. *Trends in Cognitive Sciences, 4*(6), 215-222.

18. Miller, E. K., & Cohen, J. D. (2001). An integrative theory of prefrontal cortex function. *Annual Review of Neuroscience, 24*(1), 167-202.

19. Laughlin, S. B., & Sejnowski, T. J. (2003). Communication in neuronal networks. *Science, 301*(5641), 1870-1874.

20. Firth, J., Siddiqi, N., Koyanagi, A., et al. (2019). The Lancet Psychiatry Commission: a blueprint for protecting physical health in people with mental illness. *The Lancet Psychiatry, 6*(8), 675-712.

21. American Psychiatric Association. (2013). *Diagnostic and Statistical Manual of Mental Disorders* (5th ed.). Arlington, VA: American Psychiatric Publishing.

22. Livesley, W. J., Jang, K. L., & Vernon, P. A. (1998). Phenotypic and genetic structure of traits delineating personality disorder. *Archives of General Psychiatry, 55*(10), 941-948.

23. Siever, L. J., & Davis, K. L. (1991). A psychobiological perspective on the personality disorders. *American Journal of Psychiatry, 148*(12), 1647-1658.

24. Wang, P. S., Berglund, P., Olfson, M., Pincus, H. A., Wells, K. B., & Kessler, R. C. (2005). Failure and delay in initial treatment contact after first onset of mental disorders in the National Comorbidity Survey Replication. *Archives of General Psychiatry, 62*(6), 603-613.

25. Thornicroft, G. (2011). Physical health disparities and mental illness: the scandal of premature mortality. *The British Journal of Psychiatry, 199*(6), 441-442.

26. McGorry, P. D., Purcell, R., Goldstone, S., & Amminger, G. P. (2011). Age of onset and timing of treatment for mental and substance use disorders: implications for preventive intervention strategies and models of care. *Current Opinion in Psychiatry, 24*(4), 301-306.

CHAPTER 2
DISPELLING THE MYTHS ABOUT MENTAL ILLNESS

"Doctor, I'm worried about my neighbor. He talks to himself sometimes, and he's acting strange. Should I be afraid?" This person's voice expressed genuine concern mixed with fear. This represents one of the most persistent and damaging myths about mental illness: that people with psychiatric conditions are inherently dangerous.

What is the reality? Individuals with mental illness are far more likely to be victims of violence than perpetrators. Only 3-5% of violent acts can be attributed to mental illness, while people with severe mental conditions are ten times more likely to be victims of violent crime than members of the general population.[1] Yet the media, including Hollywood and news outlets, continue to perpetuate the image of the "dangerous mentally ill person"—"they must be crazy"—creating fear where compassion should exist. Too often the media and elected officials like to immediately assign blame before any facts are available. This further stigmatizes individuals with mental health conditions.

MYTH #1: MENTAL ILLNESS IS A SIGN OF WEAKNESS

One of the most damaging myths is that mental illness suggests a personal failing or lack of strength. People will say: "He (or she) just needs to try harder," or "pray more," or "think more positive thoughts." I have also heard people share what works for them, like exercising more or eating better. While these things may work for people without mental conditions, they can often reinforce the feelings of failure that individuals with mental illness experience when they hear these casual suggestions.

The truth is that mental illness can affect anyone, regardless of their strength, intelligence, or character.[2] In fact, some of the strongest people I have worked with have struggled for years with mental conditions and managed to somehow maintain employment and relationships. Historically, there are many examples of notable figures with mental health challenges, such as Abraham Lincoln and John F. Kennedy.[3] Winston Churchill called his depression "the black dog."[4] More recently, athletes like Michael Phelps and Simone Biles have talked openly about their struggles. All of these individuals, by any measure, would be considered among the strongest of the strong.

Would anyone tell a person with diabetes to "just make more insulin" or suggest that an individual with a broken leg should "just walk it off"? So why do we apply impossible standards to individuals with mental illness? Since research has established mental illnesses to be disorders of the brain—thus medical in nature—we should be encouraging medical interventions. These aren't moral failings requiring moral correction.

MYTH #2: PEOPLE WITH MENTAL ILLNESS ARE DANGEROUS AND UNPREDICTABLE

Associating mental illness with violence is one of the most persistent and harmful stereotypes in our society. News reports overemphasize perpetrators of violence as likely or possibly mentally ill, often without any knowledge about the individual.[5] It is assumed that the individual must be "crazy" or "deranged." This ignores the fact that the vast majority of people with mental illness never commit violent acts. It's similar to when a plane crashes, killing its passengers and crew. This is tragic and scary, but the fact remains that the drive to the airport is still far riskier than the plane flight itself, statistically.

Multiple large-scale studies show that people with mental illness account for only 3-5% of violent crimes.[6] The strongest predictors of violence are substance abuse, history of trauma, and access to weapons.[7]

People with mental illness are ten times more likely to be victims of violent crime, not perpetrators.[8] They are often targets because of their social isolation, financial vulnerability, and housing challenges. Stigma only worsens the likelihood that individuals will actually seek help, which amplifies their symptoms and disability.

MYTH #3: MENTAL ILLNESS IS RARE

Another misconception is that mental illness only affects a small percentage of the population. To the contrary, nearly one in four American adults experiences some form of mental illness in any given year.[9] Over the course of a lifetime, nearly half of all Americans will meet criteria for a mental health disorder.[10] I have always said to my fellow physicians and medical providers who didn't go into psychiatry that half of the patients they see would have psychiatric needs.

When you add in other mental health challenges such as significant stress, losses, grief, life transitions, and the inevitable relationship difficulties, everyone will be impacted by mental struggles. The difference is that those with mental illness typically experience more severe symptoms with greater duration and impact on function.

With prevalence comes a silver lining: we have extensive research showing effective evidence-based treatments. The conditions showing the highest rates of success are mood and anxiety disorders such as major depression, bipolar disorder, and generalized anxiety disorder.[11]

MYTH #4: MENTAL ILLNESS IS PERMANENT AND UNTREATABLE

Another belief is that mental illness is a life sentence of suffering. The media often portrays worst-case scenarios, cementing our views about mental illness being chronic and disabling. While this may sometimes be true of the most severe cases, such as schizophrenia, it doesn't do justice to more treatable conditions such as mood disorders and substance use disorders. Even schizophrenia has a 20-30% recovery rate if treated early and aggressively.[12] Eighty percent of people with depression will respond to treatment.[13] Bipolar disorder, when treated properly with medication and therapy, allows many people to live stable, productive lives.[14]

The essential factors for improved outcomes include early and consistent interventions, social supports, and patient education about their condition. I would also add that the more insight the individual has into their condition, the better their outcomes will be. This is yet another reason why reducing stigma is so critical.

MYTH #5: MEDICATION IS ALWAYS NECESSARY (OR NEVER NECESSARY)

I often encounter two extremes: either individuals believe that medications are harmful and should be avoided at all costs, or that medications always have to be taken lifelong. Like everything else in life, the truth lies somewhere in the middle. One of the key factors has to do with severity. In the case of schizophrenia, severe bipolar disorder, and sometimes major depressive disorder, medications will be lifelong. In the case of milder forms of depression and anxiety disorders, individuals may only need medications temporarily or intermittently.[15]

With the introduction of Transcranial Magnetic Stimulation (TMS), which is the only form of biological treatment that has "durability," successful treatment cases can result in individuals with major depression (even severe forms) experiencing months or years of remission with or without medications.[16] TMS is one of the most well-studied treatments for depression of all time. Even more surprising, it's a treatment that hasn't shown any long-term side effects, making it among the safest.[17]

The goal of mental health interventions is to use the lowest effective doses and least amount of medications possible. This does require skilled clinicians attuned to the latest and most effective treatments available. I call it "custom work"—no one size fits all.

MYTH #6: CHILDREN CAN'T HAVE MENTAL ILLNESS

Another prevailing belief is that mental illness doesn't affect children or that their mental health issues are just "phases" that they will outgrow. While it is true that the transition from childhood to adulthood can be challenging, mental illness can begin at any age. Misconceptions about this can delay needed treatment and interventions, worsening outcomes.

ADHD, anxiety disorders, depression, autism spectrum disorders, and other mood disorders can emerge in childhood. About 20% of children and adolescents experience a mental health disorder, and half of all lifetime mental health conditions begin by age 14.[18]

Early intervention is particularly important for the young developing brain, as treatments may be more effective and can prevent symptoms from worsening over time. The younger brain has more neuroplasticity, meaning it is more amenable to change.[19] In addition, we can teach coping skills that will provide lifelong benefit. I have often quipped that we don't typically learn coping skills in school and sometimes not at home. We certainly don't learn them through osmosis. It's something we all have to seek out.

MYTH #7: MENTAL ILLNESS IS CAUSED BY BAD PARENTING

I was trained in medicine and psychiatry in the 1980s. It was a time when the biological revolution was taking place in psychiatry. In fact, there were far fewer programs available that taught true biological psychiatry. We were coming out of a long period of Freudian psychoanalytic psychotherapy. This was highly influential, dating back decades. It influenced Hollywood and many academics. The idea that parents played a central role in mental illness development was pervasive and damaging.[20] It laid the groundwork for years of stigma and misunderstanding. This created generations of adults feeling guilty about their children's mental illness. I am thankful that I was able to go to a training program that broke that mold. Data became king, where research was front and center. The famous line from my psychiatry department chair George Winokur, MD, when presented with an argument about mental illness was: "Show me the data." Nothing could have been more relevant then, as it is now.

With that said, the family environment is not inconsequential. Our life experiences do matter. Mental illness can emerge from loving, supportive families as well as abusive and neglectful ones. The abusive environments can create more severity and complexity, and this can't be understated.[21]

A takeaway is that parents can control their response to their child's mental health needs. Providing support, seeking appropriate treatment, reducing blame and criticism, and providing positive reinforcement and hope can improve outcomes. Just like I learned on the first day of medical school: "Do no harm."

THE REAL DANGER OF STIGMA

There are measurable consequences to stigma. It prevents individuals from seeking help and leads to discrimination in employment and housing. It also contributes to social isolation, worsening symptoms.[22]

Research shows that stigma is often more destructive than the mental illness itself.[23] People develop "self-stigma," internalizing negative stereotypes and believing they are internally flawed, leading to hopelessness. This creates a vicious cycle.[24]

The stigma of mental illness can also lead to violent acts toward the mentally ill, especially the most vulnerable—the homeless population. The media can capitalize on stigma, further worsening deep-seated misinformation about mental illness. The court system itself has often been overly biased against individuals with mental illness, making them vulnerable to excessive incarceration.[25] They are rarely able to afford proper representation and have to resort to plea deals under pressure with few options.

BUILDING UNDERSTANDING AND COMPASSION

The solution to solving the stigma problem is education, personal contact, and ultimately understanding.[26] This book is dedicated to educating about the medical nature of mental illness and providing information about effective treatments. I will provide realistic solutions used in everyday examples of the types of mental illnesses present in our society. I will illustrate this with stories of individuals that are typical for various psychiatric conditions. Although they are fictitious, they will represent the real-life people I have seen for many years.

You will see that mental illness isn't entirely hopeless. Many biological and psychological interventions are very successful. Mental illness is not something to fear. It is not a weakness.

As you move forward in subsequent chapters, I hope you will develop more compassion as you better understand the causes, interventions, and outcomes of many types of mental illness. After all, we are just taking a deeper dive into humanity in all its colors, successes, and failures.

FOOTNOTES

1. Fazel, S., Gulati, G., Linsell, L., Geddes, J. R., & Grann, M. (2009). Schizophrenia and violence: systematic review and meta-analysis. *PLoS Medicine, 6*(8), e1000120. ↩

2. Kessler, R. C., Berglund, P., Demler, O., Jin, R., Merikangas, K. R., & Walters, E. E. (2005). Lifetime prevalence and age-of-onset distributions of DSM-IV disorders in the National Comorbidity Survey Replication. *Archives of General Psychiatry, 62*(6), 593-602. ↩

3. Shenk, J. W. (2005). *Lincoln's Melancholy: How Depression Challenged a President and Fueled His Greatness*. Boston: Houghton Mifflin. ↩

4. Storr, A. (1991). Churchill's black dog and other phenomena of the human mind. *Psychiatric Bulletin, 15*(9), 544-545. ↩

5. McGinty, E. E., Webster, D. W., & Barry, C. L. (2013). Effects of news media messages about mass shootings on attitudes toward persons with serious mental illness and public support for gun control policies. *American Journal of Psychiatry, 170*(5), 494-501. ↩

6. Swanson, J. W., McGinty, E. E., Fazel, S., & Mays, V. M. (2015). Mental illness and reduction of gun violence and suicide: bringing epidemiologic research to policy. *Annals of Epidemiology, 25*(5), 366-376. ↩

7. Elbogen, E. B., & Johnson, S. C. (2009). The intricate link between violence and mental disorder: results from the National Epidemiologic

Survey on Alcohol and Related Conditions. *Archives of General Psychiatry, 66*(2), 152-161. ↩

8. Maniglio, R. (2009). Severe mental illness and criminal victimization: a systematic review. *Acta Psychiatrica Scandinavica, 119*(3), 180-191. ↩

9. National Institute of Mental Health. (2023). Mental Illness. Retrieved from https://www.nimh.nih.gov/health/statistics/mental-illness ↩

10. Kessler, R. C., Berglund, P., Demler, O., Jin, R., Merikangas, K. R., & Walters, E. E. (2005). Lifetime prevalence and age-of-onset distributions of DSM-IV disorders in the National Comorbidity Survey Replication. *Archives of General Psychiatry, 62*(6), 593-602. ↩

11. Cuijpers, P., Karyotaki, E., Weitz, E., Andersson, G., Hollon, S. D., & van Straten, A. (2014). The effects of psychotherapies for major depression in adults on remission, recovery and improvement: a meta-analysis. *Journal of Affective Disorders, 159*, 118-126. ↩

12. Jääskeläinen, E., Juola, P., Hirvonen, N., et al. (2013). A systematic review and meta-analysis of recovery in schizophrenia. *Schizophrenia Bulletin, 39*(6), 1296-1306. ↩

13. Trivedi, M. H., Rush, A. J., Wisniewski, S. R., et al. (2006). Evaluation of outcomes with citalopram for depression using measurement-based care in STAR*D: implications for clinical practice. *American Journal of Psychiatry, 163*(1), 28-40. ↩

14. Fountoulakis, K. N., Vieta, E., Young, A., et al. (2017). The International College of Neuropsychopharmacology (CINP) treatment guidelines for bipolar disorder in adults (CINP-BD-2017), part 4: unmet needs in the treatment of bipolar disorder and recommendations for future research. *International Journal of Neuropsychopharmacology, 20*(2), 196-205. ↩

15. National Institute for Health and Care Excellence. (2022). Depression in adults: treatment and management. NICE guideline [NG222]. Retrieved from https://www.nice.org.uk/guidance/ng222 ↩

16. Dunner, D. L., Aaronson, S. T., Sackeim, H. A., et al. (2014). A multisite, naturalistic, observational study of transcranial magnetic stimulation for patients with pharmacoresistant major depressive disorder: durability of benefit over a 1-year follow-up period. *Journal of Clinical Psychiatry, 75*(12), 1394-1401. ↩

17. Rossi, S., Hallett, M., Rossini, P. M., Pascual-Leone, A., & Safety of TMS Consensus Group. (2009). Safety, ethical considerations, and application guidelines for the use of transcranial magnetic stimulation in clinical practice and research. *Clinical Neurophysiology, 120*(12), 2008-2039. ↩

18. Merikangas, K. R., He, J. P., Burstein, M., et al. (2010). Lifetime prevalence of mental disorders in U.S. adolescents: results from the National Comorbidity Survey Replication–Adolescent Supplement (NCS-A). *Journal of the American Academy of Child & Adolescent Psychiatry, 49*(10), 980-989. ↩

19. Andersen, S. L. (2003). Trajectories of brain development: point of vulnerability or window of opportunity? *Neuroscience & Biobehavioral Reviews, 27*(1-2), 3-18. ↩

20. Harrington, A. (2019). *Mind Fixers: Psychiatry's Troubled Search for the Biology of Mental Illness*. New York: W. W. Norton & Company. ↩

21. Teicher, M. H., & Samson, J. A. (2016). Annual research review: enduring neurobiological effects of childhood abuse and neglect. *Journal of Child Psychology and Psychiatry, 57*(3), 241-266. ↩

22. Corrigan, P. W., Druss, B. G., & Perlick, D. A. (2014). The impact of mental illness stigma on seeking and participating in mental health care. *Psychological Science in the Public Interest, 15*(2), 37-70. ↩

23. Livingston, J. D., & Boyd, J. E. (2010). Correlates and consequences of internalized stigma for people living with mental illness: a systematic review and meta-analysis. *Social Science & Medicine, 71*(12), 2150-2161. ↩

24. Corrigan, P. W., Larson, J. E., & Rüsch, N. (2009). Self-stigma and the "why try" effect: impact on life goals and evidence-based practices. *World Psychiatry, 8*(2), 75-81. ↩

25. Prins, S. J. (2014). Prevalence of mental illnesses in US state prisons: a systematic review. *Psychiatric Services, 65*(7), 862-872. ↩

26. Corrigan, P. W., Morris, S. B., Michaels, P. J., Rafacz, J. D., & Rüsch, N. (2012). Challenging the public stigma of mental illness: a meta-analysis of outcome studies. *Psychiatric Services, 63*(10), 963-973. ↩

CHAPTER 3
UNDERSTANDING PERSONALITY TYPES AND MENTAL HEALTH

Personality is not a mental illness, but it significantly influences how mental health conditions present and respond to treatment. Personality disorders that are classified in the DSM-5 (Diagnostic and Statistical Manual of Mental Disorders, 5th Edition) meet the core criteria for mental disorders or illnesses. They meet these criteria because they have an enduring pattern of inner experience and behavior that deviates markedly from the expectations of the individual's culture. They are inflexible and pervasive across a broad range of personal and social situations, leading to distress or impairment in social, occupational, and other areas of important functioning. Personality disorders are stable and of long duration, with an onset starting around adolescence or early adulthood. The DSM-5 classifies personality disorders into Clusters A, B, and C. Cluster A is generally referred to as odd or eccentric. Cluster B is characterized as dramatic, emotional, or erratic, and Cluster C as anxious or fearful. See below for the breakdown and specific types.

DSM-5 PERSONALITY DISORDER CLUSTERS

Cluster A: Odd/Eccentric

Disorder	Key Characteristics
Paranoid Personality Disorder	Pervasive distrust and suspicion of others, belief that others are exploiting or deceiving them, reluctance to confide in others, reading hidden meanings into benign remarks, bearing grudges, and quick to counterattack
Schizoid Personality Disorder	Detachment from social relationships, limited range of emotional expression, indifference to praise or criticism, lack of interest in social or sexual relationships, preference for solitary activities, and emotional coldness
Schizotypal Personality Disorder	Magical thinking, unusual perceptual experiences, odd beliefs, odd thinking and speech, suspiciousness, limited social relationships, excessive social anxiety, and inappropriate affect

Cluster B: Dramatic/Emotional

Disorder	Key Characteristics
Antisocial Personality Disorder	Persistent pattern of violating others' rights, lack of remorse, deceitfulness, impulsivity, irritability, and aggressive behavior
Borderline Personality Disorder	Intense fear of abandonment, unstable relationships, unstable self-image, impulsive behaviors, emotional dysregulation, chronic emptiness, and identity disturbance
Histrionic Personality Disorder	Excessive emotionality, need for attention, theatrical behavior, suggestibility, easily influenced, self-centeredness, and shallow emotions
Narcissistic Personality Disorder	Grandiose sense of self-importance, preoccupation with fantasies of success, need for excessive admiration, sense of entitlement, interpersonally exploitative, and lack of empathy

Cluster C: Anxious/Fearful

Disorder	Key Characteristics
Avoidant Personality Disorder	Social inhibition, feelings of inadequacy, hypersensitivity to negative evaluation, avoidance of occupational activities that involve interpersonal contact, avoidance of social situations, reluctance to take personal risks, and fear of embarrassment
Dependent Personality Disorder	Difficulty making decisions without excessive advice from others, need for others to assume responsibility for major decisions, difficulty disagreeing with others, difficulty initiating projects independently, excessive lengths to obtain support and nurturance, and discomfort when alone
Obsessive-Compulsive Personality Disorder	Preoccupation with orderliness and control, perfectionism interfering with task completion, excessive devotion to work, inability to discard worn-out objects, reluctance to delegate tasks, miserly spending habits, and rigidity in thinking and behavior

Source: American Psychiatric Association. (2013). Diagnostic and Statistical Manual of Mental Disorders (5th ed.). Arlington, VA: American Psychiatric Publishing.

The course of personality disorders is generally chronic, but the severity of symptoms for some personality disorders may weaken with age, usually in the 40s and 50s.[1] While the outcomes vary, Borderline PD seems to lessen with age, whereas Antisocial PD and Schizotypal PD seem to persist.[2]

TREATMENT APPROACHES

There are no specific medications used to treat personality disorders. The gold standard is various forms of psychotherapy.[3] Medications may be used to target comorbid symptoms such as depression, anxiety, mood instability, and impulsivity. However, medications generally will be considered more supplemental.

The response to treatment is highly dependent on the patient's motivation to change, the severity of the disorder, and the presence of co-occurring mental health conditions. Cluster A and Antisocial Personality Disorder (sometimes referred to as sociopathy) are often less likely to seek or remain in treatment compared to Borderline Personality Disorder or Cluster C disorders.[4] Half of Borderline Personality Disorder patients will not respond to psychotherapy.[5]

DISTINGUISHING OCD FROM OBSESSIVE-COMPULSIVE PERSONALITY DISORDER

As a key distinction, Obsessive-Compulsive Disorder (OCD) is an episodic disorder (although it can be chronic) characterized by intrusive thoughts (or obsessions) resulting in compulsive behaviors. OCD tends to be disabling and nonproductive. In contrast, Obsessive-Compulsive Personality Disorder is a lifelong, pervasive, and rigid disorder. It tends to make someone very productive but hard to have a relationship with.

People with OCD tend to be distressed by their symptoms and recognize them as irrational. They may be embarrassed and won't share their symptoms unless asked. Mental health professionals will often miss OCD due to a failure to inquire.[6] People with Obsessive-Compulsive Personality Disorder are generally not distressed by their traits and often take pride in their orderliness. They may cause more distress to those around them.

OCD involves true obsessions (distressing thoughts) and compulsions (actions to relieve the distress). Obsessive-Compulsive Personality Disorder involves a chronic preoccupation with order, rules, and perfectionism, but not necessarily the intrusive, anxiety-driven obsessions and compulsions of OCD.

With people who have OCD, there is a large variety of intrusive thoughts and compulsions that are possible. Compulsions can even involve mental gymnastics such as counting in one's head, replaying a past event or memory, overanalyzing a thought or philosophical issue, or thinking a "good" or "safe" thought to cancel out a bad thought. The key feature is having irrational intrusive thoughts followed by some compulsion to relieve the anxiety associated with them. I will discuss the treatment of OCD in a later chapter. It is important to understand the distinction between OCD and Obsessive-Compulsive Personality Disorder.

COMMON PERSONALITY DISORDERS IN CLINICAL SETTINGS

Personality disorders that tend to come to the attention of mental health professionals include Borderline Personality Disorder and Antisocial Personality Disorder. Due to the fact that individuals with Borderline PD tend to engage in recurrent self-harm acts, they end up in a psychiatric hospital frequently. They are the most common personality disorders seen in an inpatient setting.[7]

Antisocial Personality Disorder tends to be a secondary problem to why individuals end up in a psychiatric facility. They have a higher likelihood of substance abuse issues and acting out. Prisons are home to many individuals with Antisocial Personality Disorder, sometimes referred to as sociopathy.[8] Antisocial personality per se has been notoriously difficult to treat or reverse. These individuals have behaviors dating back to childhood with a disregard for and violation of the rights of others. They lack any sort of moral compass or empathy for others. They lack any guilt or remorse for their often egregious actions and crimes. This is why many find themselves locked behind bars for many years.

Other personality disorders are more likely seen in the community and are people we come across in everyday life. Narcissistic Personality Disorder is characterized by grandiosity, a need for admiration, and like Antisocial PD, a lack of empathy.[9]

The remaining personality disorders tend to exist more in the shadows and are more withdrawn or aloof, except for Histrionic Personality Disorder, which exhibits excessive attention-seeking and drama.

KEY DISTINCTIONS IN TREATMENT

The distinction between personality disorders and other mental illnesses is an important one. Whereas personality disorders are treated almost exclusively with psychotherapy, other mental illnesses tend to be treated more with biological treatments such as medications, Transcranial Magnetic Stimulation (TMS), and ECT. Some would argue they are more biological in nature. However, personality disorders are very entrenched and have potential genetic origins as well and are, in a sense, "biological."[10] Psychiatrists are trained to make these distinctions in order to identify the best, most-likely-to-work treatments. I call it "custom work," as each individual may not respond predictably to each treatment approach.

FOOTNOTES

1. Zanarini, M. C., Frankenburg, F. R., Reich, D. B., & Fitzmaurice, G. (2012). Attainment and stability of sustained symptomatic remission and recovery among patients with borderline personality disorder and axis II comparison subjects: a 16-year prospective follow-up study. *American Journal of Psychiatry, 169*(5), 476-483. ↩

2. Skodol, A. E. (2008). Longitudinal course and outcome of personality disorders. *Psychiatric Clinics of North America, 31*(3), 495-503. ↩

3. Bateman, A. W., Gunderson, J., & Mulder, R. (2015). Treatment of personality disorder. *The Lancet, 385*(9969), 735-743. ↩

4. Gunderson, J. G., & Links, P. S. (2014). *Handbook of Good Psychiatric Management for Borderline Personality Disorder*. Washington, DC: American Psychiatric Publishing. ↩

5. Cristea, I. A., Gentili, C., Cotet, C. D., Palomba, D., Barbui, C., & Cuijpers, P. (2017). Efficacy of psychotherapies for borderline personality disorder: a systematic review and meta-analysis. *JAMA Psychiatry, 74*(4), 319-328. ↩

6. Glazier, K., Swing, M., & McGinn, L. K. (2015). Half of obsessive-compulsive disorder cases misdiagnosed: vignette-based survey of primary care physicians. *Journal of Clinical Psychiatry, 76*(6), e761-e767. ↩

7. Zimmerman, M., Rothschild, L., & Chelminski, I. (2005). The prevalence of DSM-IV personality disorders in psychiatric outpatients. *American Journal of Psychiatry, 162*(10), 1911-1918. ↩

8. Fazel, S., & Danesh, J. (2002). Serious mental disorder in 23,000 prisoners: a systematic review of 62 surveys. *The Lancet, 359*(9306), 545-550. ↩

9. Ronningstam, E. (2009). Narcissistic personality disorder: facing DSM-V. *Psychiatric Annals, 39*(3), 111-121. ↩

10. Livesley, W. J., Jang, K. L., & Vernon, P. A. (1998). Phenotypic and genetic structure of traits delineating personality disorder. *Archives of General Psychiatry, 55*(10), 941-948. ↩

PART II

STORIES FROM THE MIND

CHAPTER 4
SARAH'S STORY – MAJOR DEPRESSION AND THE WEIGHT OF SADNESS

Sarah first came to my office on a gray February morning, and she seemed to carry the weight of that overcast sky in her posture. At 34, she was a successful marketing manager who had built an impressive career, owned a beautiful home, and maintained close friendships. From the outside, her life looked enviable. But Sarah hadn't felt genuinely happy in over two years.

"I don't understand what's wrong with me," she said, her voice barely above a whisper. "I have everything I should want, but I feel like I'm drowning. I wake up exhausted even after sleeping ten hours. I used to love reading, hiking, cooking elaborate meals for friends. Now I can barely get through a workday without wanting to hide under my desk."

Sarah's story illustrates one of the most misunderstood aspects of major depression: it's not about life circumstances. Depression is a medical condition that can affect anyone, regardless of their external success or apparent reasons for happiness.

THE FACE OF DEPRESSION

When most people think of depression, they imagine someone who looks obviously sad—crying, withdrawn, disheveled. Sarah didn't fit this stereotype. She still showed up to work impeccably dressed, met her deadlines, and maintained a pleasant demeanor with colleagues. Her depression was largely invisible to others, which made it even more confusing and isolating for her.

"People keep telling me I should be grateful for what I have," Sarah explained. "They suggest I take a vacation, try yoga, or just 'think positive.' If I hear one more person say I need to count my blessings, I might scream. Don't they think I've tried that? Don't they think I want to feel better?"

This is the cruel paradox of depression: it strips away your ability to experience pleasure or satisfaction from the very things that used to bring you joy. The technical term is "anhedonia"—the inability to feel pleasure in activities that were once enjoyable. It's not that Sarah didn't appreciate her job, her home, or her friends intellectually. Her brain simply couldn't generate the positive emotions that normally accompany these experiences.

UNDERSTANDING THE BIOLOGICAL REALITY

Depression involves measurable changes in brain structure and function. Modern brain imaging shows decreased activity in regions responsible for pleasure, motivation, and emotional regulation.[1] Neurotransmitter systems—particularly serotonin, norepinephrine, and dopamine—become dysregulated. Stress hormones like cortisol remain chronically elevated, affecting everything from sleep patterns to immune function.[2]

Sarah's symptoms weren't signs of weakness or ingratitude—they were symptoms of a medical condition affecting her brain's ability to function normally. Just as diabetes involves the pancreas's inability to produce adequate insulin, depression involves the brain's inability to maintain normal mood regulation.

The hereditary component was evident in Sarah's family history. Her mother had experienced several episodes of depression throughout Sarah's childhood, though it was never discussed openly. Her maternal grandmother had what family members called "nervous problems" and spent periods in what was then called a sanitarium. This genetic predisposition didn't doom Sarah to depression, but it increased her vulnerability.[3]

THE ONSET AND PROGRESSION

Sarah's depression didn't begin suddenly. Like many people, she experienced a gradual slide that was initially easy to dismiss. It started about six months after a relationship ended—not a devastating breakup, just the natural conclusion of a relationship that wasn't working for either person.

"At first, I thought I was just adjusting to being single again," Sarah recalled. "I expected to feel sad for a while. But weeks turned into months, and instead of feeling better, I felt worse. Colors seemed duller. Food lost its taste. I started canceling plans with friends because the thought of pretending to be cheerful felt exhausting."

The insidious nature of depression's onset is common. Unlike a broken bone or sudden illness, depression often creeps in gradually, making it difficult to pinpoint when normal sadness crosses the line into clinical depression. Sarah spent months attributing her symptoms to temporary stress, seasonal changes, or normal life transitions.

THE IMPACT ON DAILY LIFE

As Sarah's depression deepened, it affected every aspect of her functioning. Concentration became difficult—she would read the same email multiple times without absorbing its content. Decision-making felt overwhelming; she once spent twenty minutes in the cereal aisle, paralyzed by the simple choice between brands.

Sleep became elusive despite constant fatigue. Sarah would lie awake for hours with racing thoughts, then sleep until noon on weekends, only to wake up feeling more tired than when she went to bed. Her appetite disappeared, and she lost fifteen pounds without trying—a change others noticed and complimented, not realizing it was a symptom of illness.

"The worst part was feeling like I was watching my life from outside myself," Sarah described. "I could see that I was withdrawing from friends, performing poorly at work, neglecting my home. I wanted to care, but I couldn't access those feelings. It was like being emotionally anesthetized."

This sense of detachment—what psychologists call "depersonalization"—is common in depression. People often describe feeling like they're going through the motions of life without really living it, as if they're actors playing themselves in a movie they don't want to be in.

THE SHAME AND SELF-CRITICISM

Perhaps the most toxic aspect of Sarah's depression was the relentless self-criticism it generated. Depression has a cruel way of convincing people that their symptoms are character flaws rather than medical symptoms.

"I kept thinking I should be stronger," Sarah admitted. "I'm an educated, successful woman. I should be able to handle this. The fact that I couldn't made me feel like a fraud, like everyone would discover I was actually weak and pathetic underneath my professional exterior."

This internal critic is one of depression's most insidious features. It takes legitimate medical symptoms—fatigue, concentration problems, anhedonia—and reframes them as personal failings. The person becomes not someone experiencing an illness, but someone who is fundamentally flawed.

Sarah's shame prevented her from seeking help for months. She worried that admitting to depression would damage her career, disappoint her family, or confirm her worst fears about herself. This is particularly common among high-achieving individuals who have built their identity around competence and success.

THE TURNING POINT

Sarah's decision to seek treatment came after what she called her "parking lot moment." After another day of struggling through work meetings while feeling completely disconnected, she sat in her car in the office parking lot and realized she couldn't remember feeling genuinely happy about anything in over a year.

"I thought about my best friend's wedding the previous month," she recalled. "I should have been thrilled for her—she found someone wonderful, the ceremony was beautiful, I gave a maid of honor speech that made everyone laugh. But I felt nothing. I was going through the motions, and everyone thought I was fine, but inside I felt completely empty. That's when I knew this wasn't normal sadness."

This moment of recognition—when someone realizes their symptoms have crossed the line from normal emotional responses to something requiring professional help—is crucial for recovery. Many people struggle with depression for months or years before reaching this insight.

THE JOURNEY TO TREATMENT

Sarah's first step was scheduling an appointment with her primary care physician, Dr. Martinez, who had known her for several years. This is often the most practical starting point, as primary care doctors can rule out medical causes of depression and provide initial treatment or referrals.

Dr. Martinez conducted a thorough evaluation, including blood tests to check for thyroid dysfunction, vitamin deficiencies, and other medical conditions that can mimic depression. She also asked detailed questions about Sarah's symptoms, family history, and recent life events.

"The relief I felt when Dr. Martinez took my symptoms seriously was overwhelming," Sarah remembered. "She didn't suggest I just needed more exercise or a better attitude. She explained that depression is a medical condition and that feeling better was possible with proper treatment."

Dr. Martinez started Sarah on a selective serotonin reuptake inhibitor (SSRI) and referred her to my practice for therapy. This combination approach—medication to address the biological aspects of depression and therapy to develop coping skills and address thought patterns—represents the gold standard for treating moderate to severe depression.[4]

BEGINNING MEDICATION

Starting antidepressant medication can be an emotional process. Many people feel conflicted about taking psychiatric medications, wondering if it means they're "weak" or if the medication will change their personality.

"I was terrified that the medication would make me feel artificial or numb," Sarah admitted. "I worried that if I felt better because of a pill, it wouldn't be the 'real' me. But Dr. Martinez explained it perfectly—she said the medication wouldn't make me happy, it would restore my brain's ability to experience happiness naturally."

This distinction is crucial. Antidepressants don't create artificial emotions; they help restore normal brain function so people can experience their authentic emotions again. It's similar to how insulin doesn't create artificial blood sugar but helps the body maintain normal glucose levels.

Sarah experienced some common side effects during the first few weeks—mild nausea, slight drowsiness, and initially decreased appetite. These typically diminish as the body adjusts to the medication. More importantly, after about six weeks, she began noticing subtle improvements.

"The first thing I noticed was that my sleep improved," Sarah reported. "I was falling asleep more easily and waking up less exhausted. Then I realized I had actually enjoyed a conversation with a coworker instead of just enduring it. The changes were gradual, not dramatic, but they felt like glimpses of my old self."

THE ROLE OF THERAPY

While medication helped stabilize Sarah's brain chemistry, therapy provided essential tools for understanding and managing her depression. We began with cognitive-behavioral therapy (CBT), which focuses on identifying and changing negative thought patterns that contribute to depression.[5]

Sarah discovered she had developed what psychologists call "cognitive distortions"—systematic errors in thinking that maintain depression. She engaged in "all-or-nothing thinking," seeing herself as either completely successful or a total failure with no middle ground. She practiced "mental filtering," focusing exclusively on negative aspects of situations while ignoring positive elements.

"I realized I had become a harsh critic of myself," Sarah reflected during one session. "If a friend was struggling the way I was, I would be compassionate and supportive. But I talked to myself with a cruelty I wouldn't show to anyone else."

Learning to identify and challenge these thought patterns became a cornerstone of Sarah's recovery. Instead of automatically accepting thoughts like "I'm a failure" or "Nothing will ever get better," she learned to examine the evidence and develop more balanced, realistic perspectives.

BEHAVIORAL ACTIVATION

Another crucial component of Sarah's treatment was behavioral activation—gradually reengaging with activities that previously brought pleasure or satisfaction. Depression creates a vicious cycle where decreased activity leads to worse mood, which leads to further withdrawal.[6]

We started small. Sarah committed to taking a ten-minute walk during her lunch break, even if she didn't feel like it. She agreed to accept one social invitation per week, even if she wasn't enthusiastic about it. She began cooking simple meals again, starting with dishes that required minimal effort.

"The key was doing things whether I felt like it or not," Sarah explained. "I waited months for motivation to return naturally, but I learned that sometimes action comes before feeling. By engaging in activities despite not feeling motivated, I gradually began experiencing small moments of pleasure again."

This approach challenges the common misconception that we need to feel motivated before taking action. In depression treatment, we often need to change behavior first, and improved mood follows.

FAMILY AND SOCIAL SUPPORT

Sarah's recovery was significantly aided by her decision to confide in close friends and family about her depression. Initially, she worried about burdening others or appearing weak, but the response was overwhelmingly supportive.

"My sister told me she had wondered if something was wrong but didn't know how to ask," Sarah recalled. "My best friend shared that she had gone through something similar after college. I realized that by being secretive about my struggles, I was missing out on support that was available all along."

Education was key to helping Sarah's support system understand how to help. Well-meaning friends initially suggested solutions like "just think positive" or "try harder to have fun." But once they understood depression as a medical condition, they learned more helpful approaches—checking in regularly without pressure, offering specific support like bringing dinner or helping with errands, and celebrating small improvements without minimizing ongoing challenges.

THE GRADUAL RETURN TO WELLNESS

Sarah's recovery wasn't linear. She experienced good days and difficult days, periods of improvement followed by temporary setbacks. This normal pattern of recovery can be discouraging if people expect steady, consistent progress.

"Around month four of treatment, I had a really bad week and panicked that I was going backwards," Sarah remembered. "But you helped me understand that recovery looks more like a staircase than an elevator—there are ups and downs, but the overall trajectory is upward."

By six months into treatment, Sarah was experiencing significant improvement. Her energy had returned, she was sleeping normally, and she could once again enjoy activities that had previously felt meaningless. Most importantly, she felt like herself again—not an artificially happy version, but her authentic self with normal emotional range.

MAINTENANCE AND LONG-TERM MANAGEMENT

One of the most important aspects of Sarah's treatment was developing a long-term maintenance plan. Depression has a recurrence rate of about 50% after a first episode, so preventing future episodes became a priority.[7]

Sarah continued taking medication for a full year after her symptoms resolved, following evidence-based guidelines for preventing relapse. She also maintained monthly therapy sessions to reinforce coping skills and monitor for early warning signs of depression.

"I learned to think of depression management like managing any chronic condition," Sarah explained. "I take medication regularly, attend therapy sessions, maintain good sleep hygiene, exercise regularly, and stay connected with my support system. It's not burdensome—it's just part of taking care of my health."

LIFE AFTER DEPRESSION

Today, three years after her initial episode, Sarah leads a fulfilling life while remaining vigilant about her mental health. She has been promoted at work, maintains close relationships, and has developed new hobbies including photography and rock climbing.

"Depression taught me things about myself and life that I never would have learned otherwise," Sarah reflected. "I'm more compassionate toward others' struggles, more aware of my own mental health needs, and more appreciative of simple pleasures. I wouldn't choose to go through it again, but I'm grateful for what I learned."

Sarah also became an advocate for mental health awareness in her workplace, helping to develop employee assistance programs and reduce stigma around seeking help. Her openness about her experience has encouraged several colleagues to seek treatment for their own mental health concerns.

KEY INSIGHTS FROM SARAH'S JOURNEY

Sarah's story illustrates several crucial points about depression:

Depression is a medical condition, not a character flaw. Sarah's symptoms had clear biological underpinnings and responded to medical treatment. Her inability to "snap out of it" wasn't due to weakness but to changes in brain function.

Depression can affect anyone, regardless of life circumstances. Sarah had many reasons to be happy, but depression isn't about external circumstances. It's about the brain's ability to experience and regulate emotions.

Treatment works, but it takes time. Sarah didn't feel better overnight, but with consistent treatment, she experienced significant improvement. The combination of medication and therapy provided the most comprehensive relief.

Support systems matter. Sarah's recovery was accelerated by confiding in friends and family who provided practical and emotional support throughout her treatment.

Recovery is possible. Despite feeling hopeless during her worst moments, Sarah achieved full recovery and now leads a fulfilling life. Her experience demonstrates that depression, even when severe, is highly treatable.

Prevention is important. Sarah's ongoing attention to mental health maintenance helps prevent future episodes and maintains her overall wellbeing.

A MESSAGE OF HOPE

If you recognize yourself in Sarah's story, please know that help is available and recovery is possible. Depression may feel overwhelming and permanent when you're in the midst of it, but it's a treatable medical condition. Millions of people have walked this path before you and emerged healthier, stronger, and more resilient.

The first step is often the hardest—acknowledging that what you're experiencing isn't normal sadness and seeking professional help. But once you take that step, effective treatments and supportive communities await. Like Sarah, you can reclaim your life and rediscover the capacity for joy, connection, and meaning that depression temporarily obscures.

Depression may be part of your story, but it doesn't have to be the end of your story.

WHAT IF MEDICATIONS DON'T HELP?

Although medications for depression have been a major breakthrough, they don't work for everyone. Research has shown that antidepressants are initially effective in approximately 55% of cases.[8] Each successive medication trial shows a significant reduction in effectiveness,9 and patients can get caught in a cycle of endless medication trials with diminishing returns.10 When several different antidepressant classes have been attempted without success, alternative biological interventions need to be considered.

TRANSCRANIAL MAGNETIC STIMULATION (TMS)

Transcranial Magnetic Stimulation, or TMS, was initially discovered in 1985 by Dr. Anthony Barker, PhD, an English medical physicist in London, England.[11] He adapted a Michael Faraday electromagnetic coil and demonstrated that surface brain cells, or neurons, could be activated externally with this device. A psychiatrist by the name of Mark George, MD, happened to be in London at the time and collaborated with Dr. Barker in the development of this new and exciting technology.[12]

TMS is now used worldwide and is one of the most extensively researched treatments for depression ever developed. Patients with depression can experience complete remission of their symptoms 30-50% of the time, and another 20-30% can achieve at least partial symptom relief.[13] These success rates are particularly impressive considering that TMS is typically reserved for patients who have already failed multiple medication trials.

TMS works through the principle of neuroplasticity. Research has shown that it can strengthen particular "circuits" in the brain anatomically by increasing the number of dendritic connections.[14] This helps restore the balance of activity in the brain circuits involved in mood and emotion. It goes beyond the idea of simply altering neurotransmitters, actually creating structural changes in neural networks.

Neuroscience has progressed extensively since the initial discovery of TMS in 1985. TMS is the only treatment for depression that has demonstrated true durability, since it works through neuroplasticity. In other words, the benefits can persist for months and even years after the TMS course of treatment ends, with or without medications.[15] Patients who may have been on medications for years can sometimes become medication-free and experience what I call "true normal"—their authentic baseline functioning without chemical assistance.

Another exciting aspect of TMS is that researchers have not discovered any long-term side effects. This is the only biological intervention for depression that can make this claim.[16] In fact, some experts believe that more treatment is better with TMS. It's like exercising the brain in key areas of low functioning—think of it as going to the gym for the brain. The most common side effects are mild and temporary, including slight scalp discomfort during treatment and occasional headaches that typically resolve quickly.

In my practice and experience, TMS is the most effective and exciting treatment I can offer. I have watched patients who struggled for years with medication after medication finally achieve relief through TMS. The transformation can be profound—not just symptom reduction, but genuine restoration of functioning and quality of life.

KETAMINE TREATMENT

Ketamine is a dissociative drug traditionally used in anesthesia that has been found to be effective for treatment-resistant depression and works remarkably quickly—often within hours rather than weeks.[17] This rapid action can be life-saving for patients in acute crisis. However, its downside is significant: the average relapse rate is 7-10 days after a single treatment.[18] It doesn't have the durability of TMS, and there is not yet enough long-term data to fully understand the consequences of repeated ketamine treatments over months or years. Research is ongoing to determine optimal dosing schedules and long-term safety profiles.

ELECTROCONVULSIVE THERAPY (ECT)

ECT has been around for a long time. It uses carefully controlled electrical stimulation to create a brief seizure while the patient is under anesthesia. By creating serial treatments over time, it successfully treats depression in about 60-80% of cases.[19] It's considered the "big gun" of depression treatments—the most powerful intervention we have for severe, treatment-resistant depression.

In terms of side effects, ECT can cause short-term memory loss over time. This is usually a function of the cumulative effects of multiple treatments, which limits how many treatments one can receive.[20] It also does not have the durability of TMS—maintenance treatments are typically needed to sustain benefits. Because it's more invasive, involving anesthesia and the induction of seizures, it would be considered a later choice when nothing else has worked.

That said, ECT has definitely saved lives and still has an important place in modern medicine. Unfortunately, it has carried significant stigma, especially thanks to Hollywood's sensationalized depiction in the famous film "One Flew Over the Cuckoo's Nest" starring Jack Nicholson. Modern ECT is vastly different from these outdated portrayals—it's performed under anesthesia with muscle relaxants, is painless, and is highly regulated with strict safety protocols.

LOOKING TO THE FUTURE

Because science is forever marching forward, I have hope that increasingly effective treatments and protocols will become available in the future. Funding such critical research impacts almost everyone—directly or indirectly, we are all touched by depression. The development of new treatment modalities, refinement of existing approaches, and better understanding of which treatments work best for which patients will continue to improve outcomes for people struggling with this devastating illness.

The key message is this: if standard antidepressants don't work for you, don't give up. Multiple evidence-based alternatives exist, and one of them may provide the relief you've been seeking. Work with a knowledgeable psychiatrist who stays current with treatment advances and is willing to consider the full range of options available. Recovery is possible, even when the path is more complicated than expected.

FOOTNOTES

1. Drevets, W. C., Price, J. L., & Furey, M. L. (2008). Brain structural and functional abnormalities in mood disorders: implications for neurocircuitry models of depression. *Brain Structure and Function, 213*(1-2), 93-118.

2. Pariante, C. M., & Lightman, S. L. (2008). The HPA axis in major depression: classical theories and new developments. *Trends in Neurosciences, 31*(9), 464-468.

3. Sullivan, P. F., Neale, M. C., & Kendler, K. S. (2000). Genetic epidemiology of major depression: review and meta-analysis. *American Journal of Psychiatry, 157*(10), 1552-1562.

4. Cuijpers, P., Dekker, J., Hollon, S. D., & Andersson, G. (2009). Adding psychotherapy to pharmacotherapy in the treatment of depressive disorders in adults: a meta-analysis. *Journal of Clinical Psychiatry, 70*(9), 1219-1229. ↩

5. Hofmann, S. G., Asnaani, A., Vonk, I. J., Sawyer, A. T., & Fang, A. (2012). The efficacy of cognitive behavioral therapy: a review of meta-analyses. *Cognitive Therapy and Research, 36*(5), 427-440.

6. Ekers, D., Webster, L., Van Straten, A., Cuijpers, P., Richards, D., & Gilbody, S. (2014). Behavioural activation for depression; an update of meta-analysis of effectiveness and sub group analysis. *PLoS One, 9*(6), e100100. ↩

7. Burcusa, S. L., & Iacono, W. G. (2007). Risk for recurrence in depression. *Clinical Psychology Review, 27*(8), 959-985.

8. Rush, A. J., Trivedi, M. H., Wisniewski, S. R., et al. (2006). Acute and longer-term outcomes in depressed outpatients requiring one or several treatment steps: a STAR*D report. *American Journal of Psychiatry, 163*(11), 1905-1917.

9. Amsterdam, J. D., Williams, D., Michelson, D., Adler, L. A., Dunner, D. L., Nierenberg, A. A., Reimherr, F. W., & Schatzberg, A. F. (2009). Tachyphylaxis after repeated antidepressant drug exposure in patients with recurrent major depressive disorder. *Neuropsychobiology*, 59(4), 227-233.

10. Rush, A. J., Trivedi, M. H., Wisniewski, S. R., et al. (2006). Acute and longer-term outcomes in depressed outpatients requiring one or several treatment steps: a STAR*D report. *American Journal of Psychiatry*, 163(11), 1905-1917.

11. Barker, A. T., Jalinous, R., & Freeston, I. L. (1985). Non-invasive magnetic stimulation of human motor cortex. *The Lancet, 325*(8437), 1106-1107.

12. George, M. S., Wassermann, E. M., Williams, W. A., et al. (1995). Daily repetitive transcranial magnetic stimulation (rTMS) improves mood in depression. *NeuroReport, 6*(14), 1853-1856.

13. Carpenter, L. L., Janicak, P. G., Aaronson, S. T., et al. (2012). Transcranial magnetic stimulation (TMS) for major depression: a multisite, naturalistic, observational study of acute treatment outcomes in clinical practice. *Depression and Anxiety, 29*(7), 587-596.

14. Croarkin, P. E., Nakonezny, P. A., & Husain, M. M. (2011). Evidence-based use of transcranial magnetic stimulation in depression. *JAMA Psychiatry, 68*(4), 331-332.

15. Dunner, D. L., Aaronson, S. T., Sackeim, H. A., et al. (2014). A multisite, naturalistic, observational study of transcranial magnetic stimulation for patients with pharmacoresistant major depressive disorder: durability of benefit over a 1-year follow-up period. *Journal of Clinical Psychiatry, 75*(12), 1394-1401.

16. Rossi, S., Hallett, M., Rossini, P. M., Pascual-Leone, A., & Safety of TMS Consensus Group. (2009). Safety, ethical considerations, and application

guidelines for the use of transcranial magnetic stimulation in clinical practice and research. *Clinical Neurophysiology, 120*(12), 2008-2039.

17. Berman, R. M., Cappiello, A., Anand, A., et al. (2000). Antidepressant effects of ketamine in depressed patients. *Biological Psychiatry, 47*(4), 351-354. ↩

18. Murrough, J. W., Perez, A. M., Pillemer, S., et al. (2013). Rapid and longer-term antidepressant effects of repeated ketamine infusions in treatment-resistant major depression. *Biological Psychiatry, 74*(4), 250-256. ↩

19. UK ECT Review Group. (2003). Efficacy and safety of electroconvulsive therapy in depressive disorders: a systematic review and meta-analysis. *The Lancet, 361*(9360), 799-808. ↩

20. Semkovska, M., & McLoughlin, D. M. (2010). Objective cognitive performance associated with electroconvulsive therapy for depression: a systematic review and meta-analysis. *Biological Psychiatry, 68*(6), 568-577. ↩

CHAPTER 5
MARCUS'S JOURNEY – BIPOLAR DISORDER AND THE ROLLER COASTER OF MOOD

Marcus was 28 when his life first spiraled completely out of control, though the warning signs had been building for years. A talented software engineer with a quick wit and infectious enthusiasm, Marcus seemed to live life at a different speed than everyone else. His colleagues admired his ability to work eighteen-hour days during project deadlines, his innovative solutions to complex problems, and his natural leadership in team settings.

What they didn't see were the periods when Marcus would crash—spending days in bed, unable to summon the energy to shower or answer his phone, convinced he was a fraud who would inevitably disappoint everyone who believed in him. The dramatic swings between these extremes would eventually lead to a diagnosis that explained everything: Bipolar Disorder Type I.

The Manic High

Marcus's first full manic episode began in March, triggered by a combination of work stress, sleep deprivation, and the excitement of launching a new product. What started as increased energy and confidence rapidly escalated into something much more concerning.

“I felt like I had discovered the secret to life,” Marcus recalled. “Everything seemed possible. I was getting maybe two hours of sleep a night, but I felt more energetic than ever. I was generating brilliant ideas faster than I could write them down. I started three different side projects, signed up for graduate school, and planned a cross-country road trip—all in the same week.”

During mania, the brain’s normal regulation systems become overactive. Neurotransmitters like dopamine and norepinephrine flood neural circuits, creating feelings of euphoria, grandiosity, and boundless energy.[1] Sleep becomes unnecessary, thoughts race faster than they can be processed, and judgment becomes severely impaired.

Marcus’s coworkers initially attributed his behavior to excitement about the product launch. His increased productivity, creative ideas, and charismatic leadership seemed like assets. But as the days passed, his behavior became increasingly erratic and concerning.

“I started interrupting meetings with what I thought were groundbreaking insights,” Marcus remembered. “I would talk so fast that people couldn’t follow my train of thought. I reorganized our entire coding system over a weekend without telling anyone, convinced I had found the perfect solution. When my manager suggested I take a few days off, I laughed and told him I had never felt better in my life.”

The grandiosity characteristic of mania led Marcus to believe he possessed special insights and abilities. He stayed up all night writing what he thought was a revolutionary business plan, sent long, rambling emails to company executives, and began making grandiose claims about his projects that had no basis in reality.

The Dangerous Behaviors

As Marcus's mania intensified, his behavior became increasingly risky and impulsive. He maxed out credit cards buying equipment for his various projects, believing he would make millions from his brilliant ideas. He drove recklessly, convinced his reflexes were superhuman. He engaged in uncharacteristic sexual behavior, pursuing multiple romantic encounters with little regard for consequences.

"Looking back, it's terrifying how poor my judgment became," Marcus reflected. "I wasn't making decisions based on logic or values—I was driven by impulses that felt incredibly compelling in the moment. I thought I was invincible, that normal rules didn't apply to me."

This impaired judgment during mania often leads to consequences that persist long after the episode ends: financial problems, damaged relationships, legal issues, or career setbacks.[2] The person experiencing mania feels euphoric and confident, but their behavior appears increasingly irrational and concerning to others.

The Crash

Marcus's manic episode lasted about three weeks before reality crashed down around him. It began when his manager placed him on administrative leave after he showed up to work claiming he had solved artificial intelligence and demanding to present his "breakthrough" to the company's board of directors.

"Suddenly, it was like someone turned off a switch," Marcus described. "All that energy and confidence just evaporated. I looked around at the chaos I had created—the debt, the confused friends, the angry emails from my boss—and I felt like I was waking up from a dream to find myself in a nightmare."

The depression that follows mania in bipolar disorder is often more severe than the depressive episodes experienced by people with major depression alone.[3] The contrast between the elevated mood and energy of mania and the subsequent crash creates a particularly devastating emotional impact.

Marcus spent the next two months in the deepest depression of his life. He couldn't work, rarely left his apartment, and struggled with feelings of shame and regret about his behavior during the manic episode. The euphoria and grandiosity were replaced by crushing self-doubt and hopelessness.

"I kept replaying everything I had done during those three weeks," Marcus recalled. "I was mortified by my behavior, terrified about my job, and convinced that everyone now saw me as unstable and unreliable. I felt like I had destroyed my life and reputation in record time."

The Path to Diagnosis

Marcus's journey to proper diagnosis took several months and involved multiple healthcare providers. His primary care physician initially treated him for depression, prescribing an antidepressant that actually worsened his condition by triggering rapid cycling between mood states.

"The antidepressant made everything more intense and unstable," Marcus explained. "I would go from deeply depressed to hypomanic within days, then crash again. It was like being on an emotional roller coaster that wouldn't stop."

This highlights a crucial point about bipolar disorder: antidepressants alone can be dangerous for people with bipolar disorder, potentially triggering mania or rapid cycling.[4] This is why accurate diagnosis is so important and why bipolar disorder is often misdiagnosed initially as major depression.

Marcus's breakthrough came when his sister Emma, who had been researching his symptoms online, accompanied him to a psychiatrist appointment. Emma provided crucial information about Marcus's behavior during the manic episode—details that Marcus had difficulty recalling clearly or felt too embarrassed to share.

"Having Emma there was essential," Marcus acknowledged. "She could describe my behavior objectively and help the psychiatrist understand the full picture. I was so focused on feeling ashamed about the manic episode that I wasn't giving complete information about my symptoms."

Dr. Rodriguez, the psychiatrist, immediately recognized the pattern of bipolar disorder and explained the diagnosis to Marcus and Emma. Rather than feeling devastated, Marcus felt relieved to finally understand what was happening to him.

Understanding Bipolar Disorder

Dr. Rodriguez explained that bipolar disorder is a chronic condition characterized by distinct episodes of mania or hypomania alternating with episodes of depression. The disorder has strong genetic components—about 70-80% heritability, meaning that people with bipolar disorder often have at least one close relative with a mood disorder.[5]

"Bipolar disorder isn't just extreme mood swings that everyone experiences," Dr. Rodriguez clarified. "The mood episodes are severe enough to significantly impair functioning and last for specific periods of time. Mania isn't just feeling really happy—it's a distinct altered state involving elevated or irritable mood, increased energy, and impaired judgment."

Marcus learned that he had Bipolar Disorder Type I, which is characterized by at least one full manic episode. Bipolar Type II involves hypomanic episodes (less severe than full mania) alternating with major depression. Both types require different treatment approaches than major depression alone.[6]

The biological basis of bipolar disorder involves dysregulation of multiple neurotransmitter systems and structural differences in brain regions responsible for mood regulation.[7] Advanced brain imaging shows altered activity in the prefrontal cortex, limbic system, and other areas crucial for emotional processing.[8]

Beginning Treatment

Treatment for bipolar disorder typically involves mood stabilizers, medications that help prevent both manic and depressive episodes. Dr. Rodriguez started Marcus on lithium, one of the most effective and well-studied mood stabilizers available.

"Starting lithium felt like a major step," Marcus recalled. "It meant accepting that I had a chronic condition that would require ongoing treatment. But Dr. Rodriguez explained that lithium doesn't just treat symptoms—it actually protects the brain and can prevent future episodes."

Research shows that lithium has neuroprotective effects, potentially preventing the brain changes associated with repeated mood episodes.[9] Studies consistently demonstrate that people with bipolar disorder who take lithium have significantly lower rates of suicide, hospitalization, and functional decline.[10]

Marcus also began therapy focused on understanding his condition, recognizing early warning signs of mood episodes, and developing coping strategies. Psychoeducation—learning about bipolar disorder—became a crucial component of his treatment.[11]

Learning to Recognize Warning Signs

One of the most important skills Marcus developed was recognizing early warning signs of mood episodes. For mania, his signals included decreased need for sleep, increased goal-directed activity, racing thoughts, and becoming more talkative than usual.

"I learned that needing less than five hours of sleep for several nights in a row is a major red flag for me," Marcus explained. "Now when that happens, I immediately contact Dr. Rodriguez and adjust my routine to promote sleep and stability."

For depression, Marcus's warning signs included social withdrawal, decreased interest in activities, fatigue, and negative thinking patterns. By recognizing these early signs, Marcus could take preventive action before full episodes developed.[12]

The Challenge of Medication Adherence

One of the biggest challenges in treating bipolar disorder is medication adherence. Many people stop taking mood stabilizers when they feel well, missing the hypomanic or manic periods that, despite their consequences, can feel appealing compared to depression or normal mood.[13]

"I definitely went through a period where I missed feeling hypomanic," Marcus admitted. "Those periods of increased energy and creativity were seductive. I wondered if the medication was making me boring or ordinary. But therapy helped me understand that those episodes came with serious costs."

Marcus learned to reframe his thinking about mood stabilizers. Instead of seeing them as limiting his potential, he began viewing them as enabling his authentic self to emerge consistently. The medication didn't change his personality—it allowed his true personality to remain stable.

Rebuilding Relationships and Career

Recovery from bipolar disorder often involves repairing damage caused during mood episodes. Marcus had to address financial problems from his manic spending, rebuild trust with colleagues and friends, and work with his employer to return to his position.

"The hardest part was facing people after my manic episode," Marcus recalled. "I was embarrassed about my behavior and worried everyone would see me as unstable. But most people were more understanding than I expected, especially when I explained that I had a medical condition and was receiving treatment."

Marcus's company had an employee assistance program that provided mental health resources and job protection for employees with medical conditions. His manager, initially confused by Marcus's behavior, became supportive once he understood the medical nature of bipolar disorder.

Developing Lifestyle Strategies

Successful bipolar disorder management involves more than medication and therapy—lifestyle factors play crucial roles in maintaining stability.[14] Marcus developed several key strategies:

Sleep Hygiene: Maintaining consistent sleep schedules became paramount. Marcus goes to bed and wakes up at the same time daily, avoids caffeine after 2 PM, and uses blackout curtains and white noise to optimize sleep quality.

Stress Management: Since stress can trigger mood episodes, Marcus learned stress reduction techniques including meditation, regular exercise, and setting boundaries at work. He practices saying no to commitments that would overwhelm his schedule.

Routine Structure: Marcus maintains consistent daily routines that provide stability and help him recognize when his mood is shifting. He tracks his sleep, mood, and energy levels daily using a smartphone app.

Social Support: Marcus joined a bipolar support group where he connected with others who understood his experiences. These relationships provided both practical advice and emotional support during difficult periods.

The Role of Creativity

Many people with bipolar disorder worry that treatment will diminish their creativity. Marcus, whose innovative thinking was valued in his career, initially feared that mood stabilizers would make him less creative or productive.

"What I discovered is that medication didn't eliminate my creativity—it made it more sustainable and productive," Marcus explained. "During hypomanic episodes, I had lots of ideas but poor follow-through. Now I generate fewer ideas, but they're better developed and I actually complete projects."

Research suggests that while mood stabilizers may slightly reduce the quantity of creative output during hypomanic periods, they improve the quality and consistency of creative work over time.[15] Many successful artists, writers, and innovators with bipolar disorder credit treatment with saving their careers and lives.

Long-term Management and Success

Five years after his diagnosis, Marcus has achieved remarkable stability. He has experienced only one mild hypomanic episode and no major depressive episodes since beginning treatment. He was promoted to a senior engineering position, bought a house, and is in a stable romantic relationship.

"Bipolar disorder is part of my life, but it doesn't define my life," Marcus reflected. "I take medication daily, see Dr. Rodriguez regularly, maintain good sleep habits, and stay aware of my mood patterns. It's become as routine as brushing my teeth."

Marcus also became an advocate for mental health awareness in the technology industry, where high stress and irregular schedules can trigger mood episodes in vulnerable individuals. He speaks openly about his experience to reduce stigma and encourage others to seek help.

Lessons from Marcus's Journey

Marcus's story illustrates several key points about bipolar disorder:

Early recognition and treatment improve outcomes. The longer bipolar disorder goes untreated, the more frequent and severe episodes become.[16] Marcus's relatively quick diagnosis and treatment helped prevent additional mood episodes.

Medication is usually necessary for stability. While therapy and lifestyle changes are crucial, mood stabilizers typically form the foundation of bipolar treatment. The brain changes associated with bipolar disorder generally require pharmacological intervention.

Bipolar disorder is manageable with proper treatment. Despite being a chronic condition, bipolar disorder can be effectively managed, allowing people to lead fulfilling, productive lives.

Support systems are essential. Marcus's recovery was aided significantly by supportive family, friends, and colleagues who learned about bipolar disorder and provided ongoing encouragement.

Education and self-awareness prevent episodes. Learning to recognize warning signs and maintain lifestyle stability helps prevent future mood episodes and hospitalizations.

Hope for Others

Marcus's story demonstrates that a bipolar disorder diagnosis, while initially overwhelming, can lead to better self-understanding and improved quality of life. With proper treatment, most people with bipolar disorder can achieve stability and pursue their goals and dreams.[17]

"If I could tell someone newly diagnosed with bipolar disorder one thing, it would be that this condition is treatable," Marcus emphasized. "Yes, it requires ongoing management, but it doesn't have to limit what you can accomplish. Some of the most successful, creative, and resilient people I know have bipolar disorder. With the right treatment and support, you can not only manage this condition but thrive despite it."

The key is accepting the diagnosis, committing to treatment, and building a strong support system. Like diabetes or any other chronic medical condition, bipolar disorder requires ongoing attention and care. But with proper management, it becomes just one aspect of a rich, fulfilling life rather than an insurmountable obstacle.

Understanding Schizoaffective Disorder: Beyond Bipolar, Distinct from Schizophrenia

While Marcus's journey with bipolar disorder illustrates the challenges of mood dysregulation, another condition often misunderstood or confused with bipolar disorder—Schizoaffective Disorder—presents a different but equally treatable clinical picture. Understanding schizoaffective disorder is crucial, as it differs significantly from both bipolar disorder and schizophrenia, yet shares features of each.

What Schizoaffective Disorder Actually Is

Schizoaffective disorder is characterized by the simultaneous presence of mood episodes (either mania/hypomania or depression) and psychotic symptoms that occur independently of the mood disturbance.[18] This distinction is critical: while bipolar disorder can include psychotic features that appear only during mood episodes, schizoaffective disorder involves psychosis that persists even when mood is stable. However, this doesn't mean schizoaffective disorder is simply schizophrenia with mood problems, as is commonly assumed.

"The diagnosis was confusing at first," explained James, a 32-year-old architect diagnosed with schizoaffective disorder five years ago. "My psychiatrist kept telling me it wasn't schizophrenia, but I had psychotic symptoms. It wasn't bipolar disorder either, because the psychotic symptoms didn't go away when my mood stabilized. It took time to understand that it was its own distinct condition."

The distinction between schizoaffective disorder and schizophrenia is significant and has important implications for treatment and prognosis. Schizophrenia is characterized primarily by psychotic symptoms—hallucinations, delusions, disorganized speech and behavior, negative symptoms like reduced emotional expression and motivation, and cognitive difficulties.[19] People with schizophrenia may experience mood changes, but these are not the primary feature of the disorder.

Schizoaffective disorder, by contrast, features prominent mood disturbances as core symptoms alongside psychosis. Importantly, individuals with schizoaffective disorder typically do not experience the pronounced negative symptoms that characterize schizophrenia—the emotional flattening, social withdrawal, and motivational deficits that often severely impair functioning in schizophrenia.[20] This is a crucial distinction that affects long-term outcomes dramatically.

Schizoaffective Disorder and Bipolar Disorder: Similarities and Key Differences

The relationship between schizoaffective disorder and bipolar disorder is closer than the relationship between schizoaffective disorder and schizophrenia, yet important distinctions exist. Like bipolar disorder, schizoaffective disorder involves significant mood disturbances. However, the presence of persistent psychotic symptoms outside of mood episodes distinguishes schizoaffective disorder from bipolar disorder with psychotic features.

"When I was first being evaluated, I thought I might have bipolar disorder like many of my symptoms suggested," James reflected. "But my psychiatrist explained that even when my mood was completely stable—not depressed, not manic, just normal—I still experienced auditory hallucinations and false beliefs that felt completely real. That was the key difference. With bipolar psychosis, the hallucinations should resolve when the mood episode resolves."

James's experience highlights a critical feature of schizoaffective disorder: the psychotic symptoms occur during mood episodes but also persist during periods of normal mood. This independent occurrence of psychosis is what defines schizoaffective disorder and requires a different treatment approach than bipolar disorder alone.[21]

The Nature of Psychosis in Schizoaffective Disorder

The psychotic symptoms in schizoaffective disorder are similar to those in schizophrenia and can include auditory hallucinations (most commonly hearing voices), visual hallucinations, delusions (false beliefs held with conviction), paranoia, and disorganized thinking. However, because schizoaffective disorder includes significant mood components, individuals with this condition often retain better insight into their condition and may experience periods of relative clarity or reduced psychotic intensity, particularly when mood is stable.

"My voices are always there, but they're louder and more commanding when I'm depressed or manic," James explained. "When my mood is stable and my medications are working well, the voices are quieter, more like background noise I can sometimes ignore. But they never completely go away, which is why I need ongoing antipsychotic medication even when my mood is fine."

This pattern—where psychotic symptoms fluctuate with mood but don't disappear entirely—reflects the unique position of schizoaffective disorder on the mental illness spectrum. It shares the persistent psychosis of schizophrenia but with the mood dysregulation of bipolar disorder, yet it remains a distinct entity with its own diagnostic criteria and treatment considerations.[22]

Treatment: The Combination Medication Approach

Unlike bipolar disorder, which is typically managed primarily with mood stabilizers, schizoaffective disorder usually requires a combination of medications targeting both the mood and psychotic components of the illness. This combination approach is essential for achieving symptom control and functional recovery.

James's treatment regimen illustrates this combination approach: "My psychiatrist started me on an antipsychotic medication to address the hallucinations and delusions, and then added a mood stabilizer to manage the depressive episodes. Neither medication alone was sufficient. I needed both working together to feel stable."

Antipsychotic medications, particularly second-generation antipsychotics, form the foundation of schizoaffective disorder treatment, addressing the persistent psychotic symptoms.[23] These medications work on dopamine and serotonin systems in the brain to reduce hallucinations, delusions, and disorganized thinking. However, antipsychotics alone typically don't adequately manage the mood symptoms, which is why mood stabilizers—similar to those used in bipolar disorder treatment—are added to the regimen.

"It took some adjustment to find the right combination," James noted. "My psychiatrist tried different medications and dosages until we found a combination that reduced my symptoms without overwhelming side effects. It was a process, but worth the effort."

Some individuals with schizoaffective disorder also benefit from antidepressants or anti-anxiety medications in addition to their antipsychotic and mood stabilizer, depending on their specific symptom profile. The key is recognizing that a single medication is rarely sufficient—the combination approach addresses the multifaceted nature of the disorder.[24]

Functional Outcomes and Quality of Life

A critical and often overlooked point about schizoaffective disorder is that individuals with this condition typically achieve higher levels of functioning than those with schizophrenia. The presence of significant mood disturbance, while challenging, does not carry the same profound impact on basic functioning that the negative symptoms of schizophrenia do.

"People assume that because I have psychotic symptoms, I must be as impaired as someone with schizophrenia," James explained. "But the absence of those negative symptoms—the emotional blunting, the complete loss of motivation—makes a huge difference. I still want things, I still feel things deeply, and I can still pursue goals even when managing my illness."

Research supports this clinical observation. While individuals with schizoaffective disorder face significant challenges, they generally maintain better social functioning, employment rates, and quality of life compared to individuals with schizophrenia.[25] The preserved capacity for emotional responsiveness and motivation, coupled with access to effective combination medication treatment, allows many individuals with schizoaffective disorder to work, maintain relationships, and pursue meaningful activities.

"Five years into treatment, I'm working as an architect, which requires creativity and attention to detail," James shared. "I've had to make accommodations—I'm more careful about stress management, I'm religious about taking my medications, and I have ongoing therapy. But these feel like manageable adjustments rather than insurmountable barriers."

The Importance of Accurate Diagnosis

Like Marcus's experience with bipolar disorder, accurate and early diagnosis is crucial for individuals with schizoaffective disorder. Misdiagnosis—either as schizophrenia or as bipolar disorder alone—can lead to inadequate treatment and worse outcomes.

"If I had been diagnosed with schizophrenia and treated only with antipsychotics, my mood symptoms would likely have worsened," James reflected. "Conversely, if I had been diagnosed only with bipolar disorder and treated primarily with mood stabilizers, my psychotic symptoms would probably have persisted at distressing levels. The accurate diagnosis meant I could get the right combination of treatments."

This highlights why comprehensive psychiatric evaluation, including detailed history-taking about the timeline and independence of psychotic versus mood symptoms, is essential for proper diagnosis.[26] Healthcare providers must carefully assess whether psychotic symptoms occur exclusively during mood episodes or whether they persist during stable mood periods—a distinction that fundamentally changes the diagnosis and treatment approach.

Living Successfully with Schizoaffective Disorder

Schizoaffective disorder is a serious mental illness, but it is eminently treatable. With accurate diagnosis, appropriate medication combination, ongoing therapy, and lifestyle management similar to what Marcus developed for bipolar disorder—including sleep hygiene, stress management, routine structure, and social support—individuals with schizoaffective disorder can achieve remarkable stability and quality of life.

"If someone is newly diagnosed with schizoaffective disorder, I'd tell them it's not a life sentence of severe impairment," James emphasized. "Yes, it requires ongoing management and medication. Yes, there will be challenges. But many of us go on to lead fulfilling lives—working, having relationships, pursuing interests. The combination medication approach, while requiring some trial and adjustment, works. You're not broken; you have a treatable medical condition."

The key is accepting the diagnosis, committing to the combination medication regimen even when symptoms improve, engaging in ongoing therapy and psychiatric monitoring, and building a strong support system. Like Marcus, individuals with schizoaffective disorder who embrace treatment often discover that proper management doesn't limit their lives—it enables them to live the lives they want.

FOOTNOTES

1. Cousins, D. A., Butts, K., & Young, A. H. (2009). The role of dopamine in bipolar disorder. *Bipolar Disorders*, 11(8), 787-806.

2. Dilsaver, S. C. (2011). An estimate of the minimum economic burden of bipolar I and II disorders in the United States: 2009. *Journal of Affective Disorders*, 129(1-3), 79-83.

3. Parker, G., Fletcher, K., McCraw, S., Futeran, S., Hong, M., & Hadzi-Pavlovic, D. (2014). Bipolar depression: prototypically melancholic in its clinical features. *Journal of Affective Disorders*, 152-154, 91-96.

4. Pacchiarotti, I., Bond, D. J., Baldessarini, R. J., et al. (2013). The International Society for Bipolar Disorders (ISBD) task force report on antidepressant use in bipolar disorders. *American Journal of Psychiatry*, 170(11), 1249-1262.

5. McGuffin, P., Rijsdijk, F., Andrew, M., Sham, P., Katz, R., & Cardno, A. (2003). The heritability of bipolar affective disorder and the genetic relationship to unipolar depression. *Archives of General Psychiatry*, 60(5), 497-502.

6. American Psychiatric Association. (2013). *Diagnostic and Statistical Manual of Mental Disorders* (5th ed.). Arlington, VA: American Psychiatric Publishing.

7. Grande, I., Berk, M., Birmaher, B., & Vieta, E. (2016). Bipolar disorder. *The Lancet*, 387(10027), 1561-1572.

8. Strakowski, S. M., Adler, C. M., Almeida, J., et al. (2012). The functional neuroanatomy of bipolar disorder: a consensus model. *Bipolar Disorders*, 14(4), 313-325.

9. Quiroz, J. A., Gray, N. A., Kato, T., & Manji, H. K. (2008). Mitochondrially mediated plasticity in the pathophysiology and treatment of bipolar disorder. *Neuropsychopharmacology*, 33(11), 2551-2565.

10. Cipriani, A., Hawton, K., Stockton, S., & Geddes, J. R. (2013). Lithium in the prevention of suicide in mood disorders: updated systematic review and meta-analysis. *BMJ*, 346, f3646.

11. Colom, F., Vieta, E., Sánchez-Moreno, J., et al. (2009). Group psychoeducation for stabilised bipolar disorders: 5-year outcome of a randomised clinical trial. *British Journal of Psychiatry*, 194(3), 260-265.

12. Perry, A., Tarrier, N., Morriss, R., McCarthy, E., & Limb, K. (1999). Randomised controlled trial of efficacy of teaching patients with bipolar

disorder to identify early symptoms of relapse and obtain treatment. *BMJ*, 318(7177), 149-153.

13. Scott, J., & Pope, M. (2002). Nonadherence with mood stabilizers: prevalence and predictors. *Journal of Clinical Psychiatry*, 63(5), 384-390.

14. Frank, E., Kupfer, D. J., Thase, M. E., et al. (2005). Two-year outcomes for interpersonal and social rhythm therapy in individuals with bipolar I disorder. *Archives of General Psychiatry*, 62(9), 996-1004.

15. Simeonova, D. I., Chang, K. D., Strong, C., & Ketter, T. A. (2005). Creativity in familial bipolar disorder. *Journal of Psychiatric Research*, 39(6), 623-631.

16. Post, R. M., Denicoff, K. D., Leverich, G. S., et al. (2003). Morbidity in 258 bipolar outpatients followed for 1 year with daily prospective ratings on the NIMH life chart method. *Journal of Clinical Psychiatry*, 64(6), 680-690.

17. Gitlin, M. J., Swendsen, J., Heller, T. L., & Hammen, C. (1995). Relapse and impairment in bipolar disorder. *American Journal of Psychiatry*, 152(11), 1635-1640.

18. Malaspina, D., Owen, M. J., Heckers, S., et al. (2013). Schizoaffective disorder in the DSM-5. *Schizophrenia Research*, 150(1), 21-25.

19. American Psychiatric Association. (2013). *Diagnostic and Statistical Manual of Mental Disorders* (5th ed.). Arlington, VA: American Psychiatric Publishing.

20. Marneros, A. (2003). Origin and development of concepts of schizoaffective disorder. *Journal of Affective Disorders*, 73(3), 199-202.

21. Lake, C. R., & Hurwitz, N. (2007). Schizoaffective disorder merges schizophrenia and bipolar disorders as one disease–there is no schizoaffective disorder. *Current Opinion in Psychiatry*, 20(4), 365-379.

22. Heckers, S., Malaspina, D., Bearden, C. E., et al. (2013). Structure of the psychotic disorders classification in the DSM-5. *Schizophrenia Research*, 150(1), 11-14.

23. Meltzer, H. Y., & Cucchiaro, J. (2008). The role of serotonin in antipsychotic drug action. In A. Newman-Tancredi (Ed.), *Antipsychotic Drugs* (pp. 239-268). New York: Springer.

24. Bauer, M. S., Wisniewski, S. R., Marangell, L. B., et al. (2006). Predictors of response to treatment in first-episode bipolar disorder in the Systematic Treatment Enhancement Program for Bipolar Disorder (STEP-BD). *Journal of Affective Disorders*, 94(1-3), 51-58.

25. Malaspina, D., Goetz, R. R., Friedman, J. H., et al. (2001). Traumatic brain injury and schizophrenia in members of schizophrenia and bipolar disorder families. *American Journal of Psychiatry*, 158(3), 440-446.

26. Lichtenstein, P., Yip, B. H., Björk, C., et al. (2009). Common psychiatric disorders share the same genetic risk factors. *The Lancet*, 373(9665), 746-748.

CHAPTER 6

DAVID'S REALITY – LIVING WITH SCHIZOPHRENIA

David was 19 when his parents first brought him to my office, though the changes had been unfolding gradually for nearly two years. A bright student who had earned a partial scholarship to study engineering, David had always been somewhat shy and introverted, but his freshman year of college marked the beginning of something far more concerning than typical teenage awkwardness.

"He's not the same person," his mother Patricia said during that first appointment, her voice tight with worry. "He came home for winter break and barely left his room. He says his roommate was poisoning his food and that the professors were sending him coded messages through their lectures. When we try to talk to him about it, he gets angry and says we're part of it too."

David sat quietly during this exchange, occasionally glancing at the corners of the room as if monitoring something only he could perceive. When I asked him directly about his experiences, his responses were guarded but revealed a frightening internal world that had diverged significantly from shared reality.

THE PRODROMAL PHASE

Like many people who develop schizophrenia, David's journey didn't begin with dramatic psychotic symptoms. His parents recalled subtle changes that started during his senior year of high school—changes they had initially attributed to normal adolescent development or stress about college.

"He became more withdrawn," his father Robert remembered. "He stopped hanging out with his friends, spent hours alone in his room. We thought he was just being a moody teenager. His grades stayed good, so we didn't push it."

This gradual onset, called the prodromal phase, is typical of schizophrenia.[1] Young people may show decreased motivation, social withdrawal, declining academic or work performance, unusual thoughts or perceptions, and changes in emotional expression—all before the emergence of frank psychotic symptoms. These early signs are often difficult to distinguish from normal adolescent behavior, depression, or substance use, which contributes to delays in diagnosis and treatment.

During his first semester at college, David's symptoms intensified. He stopped attending classes regularly, convinced that other students were talking about him and planning to harm him. He began staying awake all night, listening to what he believed were voices coming through the ventilation system in his dorm room. He covered his laptop camera with tape, certain that "they" were watching him.

"I tried to tell my roommate about what was happening, but he just looked at me like I was crazy," David recalled years later. "So I stopped talking about it. But the voices didn't stop, and the feeling that I was being watched only got worse."

THE FIRST BREAK

David's first full psychotic break occurred in late February of his freshman year. Campus security found him in the library at 3 AM, having dismantled several computers because he believed they contained surveillance equipment monitoring his thoughts. When officers approached him, David became agitated and claimed they were government agents sent to silence him because he had discovered "the truth."

His parents received a call from the university's dean of students. David was being transported to the emergency room for a psychiatric evaluation. He would not be returning to campus that semester.

"That phone call changed everything," Patricia said. "We drove three hours to get to him, not knowing what we were going to find. When we saw him in the hospital, he looked at us with such suspicion and fear. Our own son thought we were his enemies."

At the emergency room, David was paranoid, agitated, and responding to internal stimuli—turning his head as if listening to voices, gesturing at empty spaces. He told the evaluating psychiatrist that he had discovered a conspiracy involving the university, the government, and his family to control his mind through electromagnetic signals. He believed his thoughts were being broadcast to others and that people could insert thoughts into his head.[2]

The emergency room physician diagnosed David with a first episode of psychosis, likely schizophrenia, and admitted him to the psychiatric unit for stabilization and further evaluation.

UNDERSTANDING SCHIZOPHRENIA

During David's hospitalization, his parents received education about schizophrenia from the treatment team. They learned that schizophrenia is a severe mental illness affecting approximately 1% of the population, typically emerging in late adolescence or early adulthood.[3]

The disorder involves three main categories of symptoms:

Positive symptoms (additions to normal experience): hallucinations, delusions, disorganized thinking and speech, and disorganized or abnormal motor behavior. These were the symptoms most evident in David's presentation—his auditory hallucinations (voices), persecutory delusions (beliefs about being poisoned and monitored), and thought broadcasting.

Negative symptoms (subtractions from normal experience): diminished emotional expression, decreased motivation (avolition), reduced speech (alogia), inability to experience pleasure (anhedonia), and social withdrawal. David's prodromal phase had featured many of these symptoms, which often emerge before positive symptoms and tend to be more persistent and harder to treat.

Cognitive symptoms: problems with attention, memory, and executive function that interfere with the ability to process information and make decisions. These symptoms, though less obvious than hallucinations or delusions, significantly impact functioning and quality of life.[4]

The biological basis of schizophrenia involves dysregulation of multiple neurotransmitter systems, particularly dopamine and glutamate, as well as structural and functional abnormalities in brain regions including the prefrontal cortex, hippocampus, and thalamus.[5] Advanced imaging studies show reduced gray matter volume and disrupted connectivity between brain regions involved in perception, cognition, and emotional processing.[6]

BEGINNING TREATMENT

The psychiatric team started David on risperidone, an atypical antipsychotic medication that works primarily by blocking dopamine receptors in the brain. The goal was to reduce his psychotic symptoms—the hallucinations, delusions, and disorganized thinking that were causing him such distress and impairing his functioning.

"The first few days were really hard," Patricia recalled. "David was convinced the medication was poison. He would hide the pills under his tongue and spit them out later. It took several days before the staff could establish enough trust for him to actually take the medication consistently."

Antipsychotic medications don't work immediately. It typically takes two to four weeks to see significant improvement in positive symptoms.[7] During David's two-week hospitalization, his parents watched anxiously for signs of improvement.

Gradually, David became less agitated and paranoid. The voices, while still present, became less commanding and frightening. He began to acknowledge, at least partially, that some of his beliefs might not be accurate—a crucial development called developing insight.

"I remember the first time David said, 'Maybe it wasn't really a conspiracy,'" Robert said. "It was tentative, and he still wasn't sure, but it was the first crack in the wall of his delusions. We felt hopeful for the first time in weeks."

However, the medication brought side effects. David gained fifteen pounds in two weeks, felt constantly sedated, and developed a tremor in his hands. These side effects—common with antipsychotic medications—would become an ongoing challenge in his treatment.[8]

THE LONG ROAD HOME

David was discharged from the hospital with appointments for outpatient follow-up, a prescription for risperidone, and instructions to continue therapy. His parents had hoped this hospitalization would be a turning point after which David would return to his normal self. The reality proved far more complicated.

"I think we believed that once David was on medication, everything would go back to how it was before," Patricia admitted. "We didn't understand that schizophrenia is a chronic condition, not something you recover from completely like a broken bone."

David moved back home with his parents. Returning to college was not feasible—his symptoms, while improved, still significantly affected his concentration, motivation, and ability to function in an academic environment. He attended weekly therapy sessions and monthly medication management appointments with a psychiatrist.

The voices never completely disappeared. Even on medication, David continued to hear voices, though they became less frequent, less commanding, and less distressing. He learned strategies in therapy to manage them—reality testing, distraction techniques, and recognizing them as symptoms rather than external reality.

"At first, the voices told me to hurt myself or accused me of terrible things," David explained. "The medication helped them become quieter, more like background noise. I still hear them, especially when I'm stressed or haven't slept well, but now I can usually recognize they're not real and ignore them."

This partial response to medication is actually quite typical. While antipsychotics are the most effective treatment we have for schizophrenia, they don't eliminate symptoms entirely for most people. Approximately 40-60% of people with schizophrenia show significant improvement with first-line antipsychotic medications, but complete remission of all symptoms is rare.[2]

MEDICATION TRIALS AND SIDE EFFECTS

Over the next two years, David tried several different antipsychotic medications. When risperidone's side effects became intolerable—particularly the weight gain and sedation—his psychiatrist switched him to aripiprazole, then olanzapine, then quetiapine. Each medication offered a different profile of benefits and side effects.

Olanzapine provided the best control of David's positive symptoms, but he gained forty pounds in three months and developed elevated blood sugar levels, putting him at risk for diabetes.[10] Aripiprazole caused severe restlessness (a side effect called akathisia) that made David feel like he needed to constantly move and pace. Quetiapine helped him sleep but left him feeling sedated and unmotivated during the day.

"Every medication was a trade-off," David reflected. "I'd get relief from the voices and paranoia, but then I'd gain weight or feel like a zombie or couldn't sit still. There were times I stopped taking the medication because the side effects felt worse than the symptoms."

This medication non-adherence is one of the biggest challenges in treating schizophrenia. Studies show that up to 50% of people with schizophrenia don't take their medications as prescribed, often due to side effects, lack of insight into their illness, or feeling better and believing they no longer need medication.[11] Each time David stopped his medication, his symptoms would gradually worsen, usually leading to a return of paranoid thoughts and increased auditory hallucinations.

After several cycles of stopping and restarting medication, David's psychiatrist suggested trying a long-acting injectable antipsychotic—a medication given as an injection every two to four weeks rather than as a daily pill. This approach helps ensure medication adherence and provides more stable blood levels of the medication.[12]

"At first, I hated the idea of getting shots," David said. "It felt like giving up control. But honestly, it's been better. I don't have to remember to take pills every day, and I don't have the option to just stop when I'm feeling frustrated with side effects. The consistency has helped keep my symptoms more stable."

THE REALITY OF NEGATIVE SYMPTOMS

While David's positive symptoms (hallucinations and delusions) improved significantly with medication, his negative symptoms proved more persistent and, in many ways, more disabling. Even with stable medication management, David struggled with motivation, social engagement, and emotional expression.

"People focus on the voices and the paranoid thoughts," David observed. "But for me, the hardest part is just feeling flat all the time. I don't enjoy things the way I used to. Even when I'm not hearing voices or feeling paranoid, it's hard to care about anything. Getting out of bed, taking a shower, calling a friend—everything feels like pushing a boulder uphill."

This constellation of negative symptoms is common in schizophrenia and often responds poorly to antipsychotic medications.[13] David's lack of motivation made it difficult to maintain routines, his diminished emotional expression created barriers in relationships, and his anhedonia (inability to feel pleasure) robbed activities of their reward value.

His parents struggled to understand these symptoms. When David spent days in his room, not answering calls from friends or showing interest in activities he once enjoyed, they initially attributed it to laziness or depression rather than recognizing it as a core feature of his illness.

"We would get frustrated with him," Robert admitted. "We'd say things like, 'You just need to try harder' or 'You can't just sit around all day.'

We didn't understand that the negative symptoms were part of his brain disorder, not a choice he was making."

COGNITIVE CHALLENGES

Beyond the positive and negative symptoms, David experienced significant cognitive difficulties that affected his ability to function independently. His working memory was impaired, making it hard to follow complex conversations or remember multi-step instructions. His processing speed was slower, requiring more time to complete tasks. His executive functioning—the ability to plan, organize, and complete goal-directed activities—was significantly compromised.[14]

These cognitive symptoms meant that returning to college-level academics was not realistic for David, despite his previously strong intellectual abilities. Even simple tasks like managing his medications, keeping appointments, and handling finances required support from his parents.

"I used to be able to juggle multiple classes, a part-time job, and a social life," David said. "Now I struggle to keep track of what day it is or remember if I already ate lunch. It's like my brain is working through fog all the time."

Cognitive remediation therapy—specialized training designed to improve cognitive functioning—helped David develop compensatory strategies. He learned to use phone reminders extensively, break tasks into smaller steps, and create structured routines to help manage his cognitive limitations.[15]

FINDING A NEW PATH

Four years after his first hospitalization, David's life looked very different from what he and his parents had envisioned. He was not in college, did not have a career, and lived in a supervised apartment with support from a community mental health program. He took medication daily via monthly injections, attended a day treatment program three times per week, and saw his psychiatrist monthly.

Yet within these significant limitations, David had found a measure of stability and purpose that seemed impossible during the chaos of his first psychotic break.

"I had to grieve the life I thought I would have," David reflected. "The engineering degree, the career, the independence—all of that went away. But once I stopped fighting against my limitations and started working within them, things got better."

David found meaning through volunteering at a local animal shelter, where he helped care for cats awaiting adoption. The work was structured, didn't require extensive social interaction, and provided a sense of purpose. The cats didn't judge him, didn't care if he was experiencing symptoms, and seemed to appreciate his gentle, patient care.

"Working with the cats gives me a reason to get up and leave the apartment," David explained. "It's something I can usually manage even when my symptoms are worse. And honestly, the cats have been better companions than most people. They don't ask questions I can't answer or expect things I can't provide."

He also connected with other people with schizophrenia through a peer support group. Unlike his previous friendships, which had fallen away when his illness emerged, these relationships were built on shared understanding of what it meant to live with severe mental illness.

"In the support group, I don't have to explain or apologize for my symptoms," David said. "Everyone there gets it. We can talk about the voices, the medication side effects, the frustration with cognitive problems—all the things that would make other people uncomfortable. It's incredibly validating."

THE FAMILY'S JOURNEY

David's illness profoundly affected his entire family. His parents had to adjust their expectations, learn to advocate within a complex mental health system, and find ways to support David while maintaining their own wellbeing.

Patricia joined a family support group through the National Alliance on Mental Illness (NAMI), where she connected with other parents of children with severe mental illness. "Meeting other families going through similar struggles was lifesaving," she said. "I realized we weren't alone, and I learned practical strategies for helping David while also taking care of myself."

The family learned about the stress-vulnerability model of schizophrenia—the understanding that while David had a biological vulnerability to the illness, environmental stressors could trigger or worsen symptoms.[16] They worked to create a low-stress home environment, with clear expectations, consistent routines, and open communication.

"We learned not to have heated arguments around David, to give him advance notice about changes in plans, and to recognize when he was becoming overwhelmed," Robert explained. "We had to find a balance between supporting him and not enabling dependency."

David's younger sister, Emily, struggled with guilt, anger, and grief over the changes in their family dynamics. Family therapy helped her process these complex feelings and develop her own relationship with her brother that acknowledged both his illness and his remaining strengths.

REALISTIC EXPECTATIONS AND MEANINGFUL PROGRESS

Six years after his diagnosis, David's life had stabilized significantly, though he continued to experience symptoms and functional limitations. He lived independently in a supervised apartment, managed his self-care with minimal assistance, maintained his volunteer work, and had developed a small but meaningful social network through his support group.

His positive symptoms were well-controlled most of the time. He still heard voices occasionally, especially when stressed or sleep-deprived, but they were manageable and no longer dictated his behavior. His paranoid thoughts had largely resolved, though he remained somewhat suspicious and guarded in new situations.

The negative symptoms persisted as his greatest challenge. David continued to struggle with motivation, emotional expression, and pleasure in activities. He needed significant structure and support to maintain his routines and functioning. His cognitive limitations meant that complex tasks remained difficult and employment in his chosen field was not realistic.

"I won't pretend David recovered completely or that everything worked out the way we hoped," I told his parents during one of our family sessions. "Schizophrenia is a serious, chronic illness. But David has made real progress. He's stable, safe, engaged in meaningful activities, and able to live with dignity despite his illness. That represents success, even if it doesn't look like the success we initially imagined."

Research supports this realistic perspective. Long-term studies show that while complete recovery from schizophrenia is rare (occurring in roughly 20-30% of cases), approximately 40-60% of people with schizophrenia achieve significant improvement in symptoms and functioning with treatment.[17] Many people, like David, reach a stable level of functioning that, while limited compared to their pre-illness baseline, allows for quality of life, meaningful relationships, and personal dignity.

THE IMPORTANCE OF EARLY INTERVENTION

One aspect of David's case that I've reflected on extensively is the delay between his first symptoms and his first treatment. The prodromal symptoms began during his senior year of high school—nearly two years before his first hospitalization. Earlier recognition and intervention during that critical period might have altered his trajectory.

Research increasingly shows that duration of untreated psychosis (DUP)—the time between onset of psychotic symptoms and initiation of treatment—significantly impacts long-term outcomes. Shorter DUP is associated with better response to medication, less severe negative symptoms, and improved functional outcomes.[18]

"If we had understood what was happening earlier, if we had gotten David into treatment during those first subtle changes, would things be different now?" Patricia wondered. "We'll never know, but I tell every parent I meet through NAMI to trust their instincts. If something seems off with their child, get them evaluated. Don't wait for a crisis."

This is why education about early warning signs of psychosis is so crucial. Many communities now have early intervention programs specifically designed to identify and treat first-episode psychosis, offering intensive, coordinated care during this critical period.[19] These programs have demonstrated improved outcomes compared to traditional treatment approaches.

LIVING WITH SCHIZOPHRENIA: DAVID'S PERSPECTIVE

When I asked David what he would want others to understand about living with schizophrenia, he thought carefully before responding.

"People think schizophrenia means you're completely out of touch with reality, that you're dangerous, that your life is over," he said. "The reality is more complicated. Yes, I have symptoms. Yes, my life is different from what I planned. But I'm still me. I still have thoughts, feelings, preferences, and goals. I still matter.

"The hardest part isn't the voices or even the paranoid thoughts—it's how people treat you when they find out you have schizophrenia. They start talking to you like you're a child, or they become afraid of you, or they just disappear from your life. The stigma is often worse than the symptoms.

"I want people to know that schizophrenia is an illness, not an identity. I'm not 'a schizophrenic'—I'm David, a person who has schizophrenia. I still have value. My life still has meaning, even if it doesn't look like what society defines as success.

"And I want other people with schizophrenia to know that even when things feel hopeless, even when the symptoms feel overwhelming, there are treatments that can help. You might not recover completely, but you can build a life worth living. It takes time, it takes support, and it takes accepting help when you need it. But it's possible."

LESSONS FROM DAVID'S JOURNEY

David's story illustrates several crucial points about schizophrenia:

Schizophrenia typically emerges gradually. The prodromal phase often begins years before the first psychotic episode, with subtle changes in functioning that are easy to miss or attribute to other causes. Early recognition and intervention can improve outcomes.

Treatment helps but rarely cures. Antipsychotic medications significantly reduce symptoms for most people, but complete remission is uncommon. Managing schizophrenia is a long-term process requiring ongoing treatment and support.

Medication side effects are a major challenge. The side effects of antipsychotic medications—weight gain, sedation, movement disorders, metabolic problems—significantly impact quality of life and medication adherence. Finding the right medication often requires trying multiple options.

Negative symptoms are often more disabling than positive symptoms. While hallucinations and delusions respond reasonably well to medication, negative symptoms (lack of motivation, flat affect, anhedonia) and cognitive symptoms often persist and significantly impair functioning.

Recovery looks different for everyone. While complete recovery is relatively rare, many people with schizophrenia achieve significant stability, symptom reduction, and quality of life with appropriate treatment and support. Success must be defined individually rather than by pre-illness standards.

Family support is crucial. Schizophrenia affects the entire family system. Education, support services, and realistic expectations help families provide effective support while maintaining their own wellbeing.

Stigma compounds suffering. Social isolation, discrimination, and negative stereotypes often cause more suffering than the symptoms themselves. Reducing stigma requires education and direct contact with people living successfully with schizophrenia.

A MESSAGE OF REALISTIC HOPE

David's story doesn't have the dramatic recovery arc of Sarah's depression or even Marcus's bipolar disorder. Schizophrenia remains one of the most challenging mental illnesses to treat, and outcomes vary widely. But David's journey demonstrates that even with persistent symptoms and significant limitations, people with schizophrenia can achieve stability, find meaning and purpose, and live with dignity.

The key is accepting the reality of the illness while maintaining hope for the future. This means:

Starting treatment as early as possible and maintaining it consistently

Finding the right combination of medications that balances symptom control with tolerable side effects

Building a strong support system including family, mental health professionals, and peers

Developing realistic goals that account for current functioning while allowing for growth

Creating structure and routine that supports stability
Challenging stigma and maintaining connection to community
Focusing on quality of life rather than complete cure

"I won't lie and say everything worked out perfectly," David reflected. "My life is harder than I ever imagined it would be. But it's still my life, and it still has value. I have people who care about me, activities that give me purpose, and hopes for the future. That's more than I had six years ago when I was in the hospital convinced the world was ending. So yes, there's hope—maybe not the hope for a complete cure, but hope for a life worth living despite this illness."

For families receiving a schizophrenia diagnosis, this realistic perspective is crucial. While the prognosis is serious and the challenges are real, treatment can help. Many people with schizophrenia, with appropriate support and care, can achieve a quality of life that seemed impossible during the chaos of first psychosis.

The goal is not perfection, but progress—measured in stability maintained, crises avoided, connections preserved, and moments of peace found amid the symptoms. By these measures, David's journey, while difficult, represents genuine success and offers hope to others walking a similar path.

FOOTNOTES

1. Addington, J., Cornblatt, B. A., Cadenhead, K. S., et al. (2011). At clinical high risk for psychosis: outcome for nonconverters. *American Journal of Psychiatry, 168*(8), 800-805.

2. Tandon, R., Gaebel, W., Barch, D. M., et al. (2013). Definition and description of schizophrenia in the DSM-5. *Schizophrenia Research, 150*(1), 3-10.

3. McGrath, J., Saha, S., Chant, D., & Welham, J. (2008). Schizophrenia: a concise overview of incidence, prevalence, and mortality. *Epidemiologic Reviews, 30*(1), 67-76.

4. Green, M. F., Kern, R. S., & Heaton, R. K. (2004). Longitudinal studies of cognition and functional outcome in schizophrenia: implications for MATRICS. *Schizophrenia Research, 72*(1), 41-51.

5. Howes, O. D., & Kapur, S. (2009). The dopamine hypothesis of schizophrenia: version III—the final common pathway. *Schizophrenia Bulletin, 35*(3), 549-562.

6. van Erp, T. G., Hibar, D. P., Rasmussen, J. M., et al. (2016). Subcortical brain volume abnormalities in 2028 individuals with schizophrenia and

2540 healthy controls via the ENIGMA consortium. *Molecular Psychiatry, 21*(4), 547-553.

7. Agid, O., Kapur, S., Arenovich, T., & Zipursky, R. B. (2003). Delayed-onset hypothesis of antipsychotic action: a hypothesis tested and rejected. *Archives of General Psychiatry, 60*(12), 1228-1235.

8. Correll, C. U., & Schenk, E. M. (2008). Tardive dyskinesia and new antipsychotics. *Current Opinion in Psychiatry, 21*(2), 151-156.

9. Leucht, S., Tardy, M., Komossa, K., et al. (2012). Antipsychotic drugs versus placebo for relapse prevention in schizophrenia: a systematic review and meta-analysis. *The Lancet, 379*(9831), 2063-2071.

10. Newcomer, J. W. (2005). Second-generation (atypical) antipsychotics and metabolic effects: a comprehensive literature review. *CNS Drugs, 19*(Suppl 1), 1-93.

11. Lacro, J. P., Dunn, L. B., Dolder, C. R., Leckband, S. G., & Jeste, D. V. (2002). Prevalence of and risk factors for medication nonadherence in patients with schizophrenia: a comprehensive review of recent literature. *Journal of Clinical Psychiatry, 63*(10), 892-909.

12. Kishimoto, T., Nitta, M., Borenstein, M., Kane, J. M., & Correll, C. U. (2013). Long-acting injectable versus oral antipsychotics in schizophrenia: a systematic review and meta-analysis of mirror-image studies. *Journal of Clinical Psychiatry, 74*(10), 957-965.

13. Kirkpatrick, B., Fenton, W. S., Carpenter, W. T., & Marder, S. R. (2006). The NIMH-MATRICS consensus statement on negative symptoms. *Schizophrenia Bulletin, 32*(2), 214-219.

14. Keefe, R. S., & Harvey, P. D. (2012). Cognitive impairment in schizophrenia. *Handbook of Experimental Pharmacology, 213*, 11-37.

15. Wykes, T., Huddy, V., Cellard, C., McGurk, S. R., & Czobor, P. (2011). A meta-analysis of cognitive remediation for schizophrenia: methodology and effect sizes. *American Journal of Psychiatry, 168*(5), 472-485.

16. Nuechterlein, K. H., Dawson, M. E., Ventura, J., et al. (1994). The vulnerability/stress model of schizophrenic relapse: a longitudinal study. *Acta Psychiatrica Scandinavica, 89*(Suppl 382), 58-64. ↩

17. Jääskeläinen, E., Juola, P., Hirvonen, N., et al. (2013). A systematic review and meta-analysis of recovery in schizophrenia. *Schizophrenia Bulletin, 39*(6), 1296-1306. ↩

18. Marshall, M., Lewis, S., Lockwood, A., Drake, R., Jones, P., & Croudace, T. (2005). Association between duration of untreated psychosis and outcome in cohorts of first-episode patients: a systematic review. *Archives of General Psychiatry, 62*(9), 975-983. ↩

19. Kane, J. M., Robinson, D. G., Schooler, N. R., et al. (2016). Comprehensive versus usual community care for first-episode psychosis: 2-year outcomes from the NIMH RAISE early treatment program. *American Journal of Psychiatry, 173*(4), 362-372. ↩

CHAPTER 7

MANDI'S STRUGGLE – BREAKING FREE FROM OCD'S GRIP

Mandi was 32 when she finally walked into my office, though she had been suffering in silence for nearly fifteen years. A successful accountant with her own small firm, Mandi appeared to have her life together—organized, detail-oriented, and professionally accomplished. What no one knew was that she was spending four to five hours every day trapped in exhausting rituals that she couldn't stop, despite knowing they made no logical sense.

"I've been too ashamed to tell anyone," she admitted during our first session, her eyes fixed on her hands. "People think I'm just really neat and organized. They have no idea that I check the stove forty times before leaving the house, or that I can't leave my office until I've touched every doorknob exactly six times, or that I spend two hours every night checking and rechecking that the doors are locked. I feel like I'm losing my mind, but I can't stop."

Mandi's story illustrates the hidden torment of Obsessive-Compulsive Disorder (OCD)—a condition that traps people in a cycle of intrusive thoughts and ritualistic behaviors that can consume hours each day and severely impair quality of life.

UNDERSTANDING OCD

Obsessive-Compulsive Disorder affects approximately 2-3% of the population, making it more common than many people realize.[1] Despite its prevalence, OCD is often misunderstood, trivialized, or confused with being highly organized or detail-oriented—what we discussed in Chapter 3 as Obsessive-Compulsive Personality Disorder (OCPD).

True OCD involves two key components:

Obsessions: Intrusive, unwanted thoughts, images, or urges that cause significant anxiety or distress. These are not simply excessive worries about real-life problems—they're irrational thoughts that the person recognizes as products of their own mind but cannot control or dismiss.

Compulsions: Repetitive behaviors or mental acts that a person feels driven to perform in response to an obsession or according to rigid rules. These compulsions are aimed at preventing or reducing anxiety or preventing some dreaded event, even though they're not realistically connected to these outcomes or are clearly excessive.[2]

The key distinction between OCD and simply being careful or organized is that people with OCD experience significant distress from their symptoms and recognize them as irrational, yet feel unable to resist performing the compulsions. The rituals provide only temporary relief before the anxiety builds again, creating an exhausting cycle.

THE HIDDEN YEARS

Mandi's OCD began when she was seventeen, shortly after she got her driver's license. She had been driving home from a friend's house when she hit what she thought might have been a pothole. A intrusive thought suddenly entered her mind: "What if that wasn't a pothole? What if I hit someone?"

"I knew it was irrational," Mandi recalled. "I had seen the pothole, felt the bump, and kept driving. But this thought just invaded my mind: 'What if you hit a person and didn't realize it? What if someone is lying in the road bleeding because of you?' The anxiety was overwhelming."

Mandi turned her car around and drove back to check. She saw nothing but the pothole. Relief flooded through her—for about five minutes. Then the doubt crept back: "But what if you missed something? What if you weren't looking carefully enough?"

She drove back again. And again. And again. By the time she finally managed to drive home, she had checked the same spot seventeen times and was shaking with exhaustion and fear.

"That was the beginning," Mandi explained. "After that, the obsessive thoughts spread to other things. Every time I locked a door, I'd wonder if I really locked it or just thought about locking it. When I turned off the stove, I'd worry it was still on and would cause a fire. The only way to reduce the anxiety was to check—but the relief never lasted."

This pattern of onset is typical for OCD, which usually begins in adolescence or early adulthood.[3] The disorder often starts with one specific obsession and compulsion, then gradually expands to encompass other areas of life. Many people, like Mandi, suffer for years before seeking treatment, often due to shame or not realizing that effective treatments exist.

THE MANY FACES OF OCD

During our initial assessment, I learned that Mandi's OCD had evolved over the years to include multiple types of obsessions and compulsions:

Contamination obsessions and cleaning compulsions: Mandi worried excessively about germs and contamination. She washed her hands dozens of times per day, often until they were raw and bleeding. She couldn't touch doorknobs, handrails, or anything in public spaces without immediately washing her hands. At home, she spent hours cleaning surfaces that were already clean.

Checking compulsions: The stove, locks, light switches, windows, appliances—Mandi checked everything repeatedly. She would lock her front door, walk to her car, then go back to check that she had actually locked it. This checking could take thirty to forty minutes before she could leave for work.

Symmetry and ordering compulsions: Items in her home and office had to be arranged in exact, symmetrical patterns. If something was out of place, Mandi experienced intense anxiety until she could fix it. She would spend an hour arranging items on her desk before she could start working.

Mental compulsions: Beyond the visible rituals, Mandi performed extensive mental compulsions. She would count in her head, repeat "safe" phrases, or review conversations to make sure she hadn't said something wrong. These mental rituals were exhausting and time-consuming, yet invisible to others.

"People would compliment me on being so organized and clean," Mandi said. "They had no idea I was drowning. I wasn't organized—I was trapped. Every day was exhausting, and I was always behind on work because so much of my time was consumed by rituals I couldn't stop."

This presentation represents moderate OCD—severe enough to significantly impact functioning and quality of life, but not so severe that Mandi was completely unable to work or care for herself. Research suggests that moderate OCD, defined as symptoms that interfere with functioning but don't completely prevent it, represents the most common severity level among people who seek treatment.[4]

THE BIOLOGY OF OCD

OCD is not a psychological weakness or a character flaw—it's a neurobiological disorder with clear brain-based mechanisms. Advanced imaging studies show that people with OCD have abnormalities in a brain circuit involving the orbitofrontal cortex, anterior cingulate cortex, and basal ganglia—areas involved in error detection, habit formation, and anxiety regulation.[5]

"Think of OCD as a false alarm system in the brain," I explained to Mandi. "Your brain's error-detection system is overactive, constantly signaling that something is wrong or dangerous even when it's not. The compulsions are your brain's attempt to 'fix' the perceived error and shut off the alarm. But because there's no actual problem to fix, the alarm keeps going off."

The neurotransmitter serotonin plays a crucial role in OCD, which is why medications that increase serotonin (selective serotonin reuptake inhibitors or SSRIs) can help reduce symptoms.[6] However, unlike depression, where lower doses of SSRIs are often effective, OCD typically requires higher doses for longer periods to see improvement.

Mandi found this neurobiological explanation liberating. "For years, I thought I was just weak or crazy," she said. "Understanding that this is a brain disorder—that there's a reason I can't just 'stop worrying about it'—helped me feel less ashamed about needing help."

BEGINNING TREATMENT

Treatment for OCD typically involves two main components: medication (usually an SSRI) and a specific type of therapy called Exposure and Response Prevention (ERP), which is a form of cognitive-behavioral therapy specifically designed for OCD.[7]

I started Mandi on sertraline (Zoloft), an SSRI that has strong evidence for treating OCD. I explained that unlike depression, where improvement might be seen in 4-6 weeks, OCD often requires 10-12 weeks at an adequate dose to see meaningful improvement. Mandi would need to be patient.

"The medication won't make the obsessive thoughts disappear completely," I told her. "But it should reduce their frequency and intensity, and make them less distressing. Most importantly, it should make it easier for you to resist the compulsions, which is where the therapy comes in."

Simultaneously, I referred Mandi to Dr. Sarah Chen, a psychologist specializing in ERP therapy for OCD. ERP would be the cornerstone of Mandi's treatment—the intervention most likely to produce lasting change.[8]

UNDERSTANDING EXPOSURE AND RESPONSE PREVENTION

During her first session with Dr. Chen, Mandi learned about the treatment that would prove most effective for her OCD: Exposure and Response Prevention (ERP).

"ERP works by breaking the cycle between obsessions and compulsions," Dr. Chen explained. "Right now, when you have an obsessive thought—like 'Did I lock the door?'—your anxiety spikes. You check the door, which temporarily reduces the anxiety. But this checking actually strengthens the OCD cycle because your brain learns: 'Checking makes me feel better, so I should check whenever I'm anxious.'"

ERP involves two key components:

Exposure: Deliberately triggering the obsessive thoughts and anxiety without immediately performing the compulsion. For Mandi, this might mean locking the door once and then walking away despite the anxiety about whether it was really locked.

Response Prevention: Resisting the urge to perform the compulsion, allowing the anxiety to naturally decrease over time without reinforcing the ritual. This teaches the brain that the feared outcome doesn't actually occur and that anxiety decreases on its own without the compulsion.

"I'm not going to lie," Dr. Chen said. "ERP is hard. You're going to have to deliberately make yourself anxious and then sit with that discomfort. It goes against every instinct you have. But it works, and the research supporting it is rock solid."

Mandi was terrified. "You want me to just... not check? To leave the house without checking the stove? What if there actually is a fire?"

"That's the OCD talking," Dr. Chen replied gently. "The likelihood of your stove causing a fire if you've turned it off once is astronomically small—the same as for everyone else who doesn't have OCD. But your brain is convinced the risk is high. ERP will help retrain your brain to accept normal levels of uncertainty."

THE ERP JOURNEY

Dr. Chen and Mandi worked together to create a hierarchy of feared situations, ranked from least to most anxiety-provoking. They would start with exposures that caused moderate anxiety and gradually work up to more challenging ones.

Mandi's first exposure exercise seemed deceptively simple: touch a doorknob in Dr. Chen's office and then sit with her hands "contaminated" for fifteen minutes without washing them.

"Those fifteen minutes felt like hours," Mandi recalled. "My anxiety was through the roof. I kept thinking about all the germs on my hands, imagining getting sick, wanting desperately to wash. But Dr. Chen sat with me, talked me through it, and kept reminding me that the anxiety would decrease if I didn't give in to the compulsion."

After about ten minutes, something remarkable happened: Mandi's anxiety began to decrease on its own. Not completely—she was still uncomfortable—but the peak had passed without her washing her hands.

"That first time my anxiety went down without me doing anything to make it go down—that was huge," Mandi said. "It proved that I didn't need the compulsion to feel better. The anxiety would pass on its own if I just waited it out."

Over the following weeks, Mandi and Dr. Chen worked through increasingly challenging exposures:

Touching multiple surfaces in public without washing hands immediately
Locking the door once and leaving without checking
Turning off the stove once and leaving the house
Leaving items on her desk slightly asymmetrical
Resisting mental counting rituals

Each exposure followed the same pattern: intense anxiety initially, followed by gradual habituation as Mandi sat with the discomfort without performing compulsions. The medication helped by taking the edge off her anxiety, making the exposures more manageable.[2]

SETBACKS AND PROGRESS

Mandi's recovery wasn't linear. There were weeks when she made significant progress, reducing her daily ritual time from four hours to ninety minutes. Then there were weeks when stress at work triggered a resurgence of symptoms and she found herself checking repeatedly again.

"I had a big audit coming up at work," Mandi explained. "The stress brought back all my checking behaviors. I felt like I was back at square one, and I was devastated."

"Setbacks are a normal part of recovery," I assured her. "OCD symptoms often worsen during stress. What matters is that you now have tools to address them. You know how to do exposures. You understand that giving in to compulsions will only strengthen the OCD in the long run."

This understanding of OCD as a chronic condition requiring ongoing management is important. While many people achieve significant improvement or even remission of symptoms, OCD often requires long-term treatment and vigilance.[10] The goal is not perfection, but rather developing skills to manage symptoms when they arise and preventing them from controlling your life.

Mandi worked with Dr. Chen to implement stress-management techniques and to recognize early warning signs that her OCD was worsening. She learned that increasing her ERP practice during stressful periods could prevent a full relapse into severe symptoms.

WHEN STANDARD TREATMENT ISN'T ENOUGH: DEEP TMS

After six months of combined medication and ERP therapy, Mandi had made progress—her daily ritual time had decreased from four hours to about two hours—but she was still significantly impaired. The obsessive thoughts remained intense, and resisting compulsions continued to require enormous effort. She was frustrated by the slow pace of improvement.

"I'm doing everything right," Mandi said during one of our sessions. "I'm taking the medication, doing the ERP exercises, but I still feel like OCD controls too much of my life. Is this as good as it gets?"

I explained that for some people with OCD, standard treatments don't provide sufficient relief. In these cases, we have additional options, including a relatively new treatment called Deep Transcranial Magnetic Stimulation (Deep TMS), specifically the BrainsWay system, which had recently received FDA approval for treating OCD.[11]

"Deep TMS is different from the regular TMS used for depression," I explained. "The BrainsWay device uses a specialized coil called an H-coil that can reach deeper brain structures, including the anterior cingulate cortex and other areas involved in the OCD brain circuit. It's non-invasive, has minimal side effects, and research shows it can significantly reduce OCD symptoms."[12]

The treatment involves daily sessions, five days a week for six weeks. During each twenty-minute session, the device delivers magnetic pulses to specific brain regions involved in OCD. Unlike medication, which affects the entire brain, Deep TMS targets the specific neural circuits that are dysfunctional in OCD.[13]

"What convinced me to try it was that it could work alongside my medication and therapy," Mandi recalled. "It wasn't replacing what I was already doing—it was adding another tool to help my brain change. And the fact that it had FDA approval for OCD specifically made me feel confident it was a legitimate treatment."

Research on Deep TMS for OCD has shown promising results. The pivotal randomized controlled trial demonstrated that approximately 38% of patients achieved clinical response with Deep TMS compared to 11% with sham treatment.[14] More recently, real-world data from twenty-two clinical sites—research that I participated in as a contributing investigator—showed that Deep TMS produced significant symptom reduction in actual clinical practice settings, with patients experiencing an average 30% reduction in OCD symptoms.[15] Even more encouraging, long-term follow-up studies have demonstrated that the benefits of Deep TMS can be sustained over time, with many patients maintaining improvement for months to years after completing the initial treatment course.[16]

The treatment appears to work by normalizing the hyperactive circuits in the brain that drive obsessive thoughts and compulsive behaviors. The H-coil's ability to reach deeper brain structures like the anterior cingulate cortex—a key region in the OCD circuit—distinguishes it from standard TMS coils.[17]

Mandi began Deep TMS treatment, attending daily sessions at a specialized clinic. "The treatment itself was straightforward," she said. "I sat in a comfortable chair while they positioned the coil over my head. I felt a tapping sensation during the magnetic pulses, but it wasn't painful. I could read or listen to music during the session."

After about three weeks of treatment, Mandi began noticing changes. "The obsessive thoughts didn't disappear, but they became less intense and less frequent," she explained. "More importantly, resisting the compulsions became easier. It was like the 'volume' of the OCD had been turned down, making the ERP work more effective."

By the end of the six-week Deep TMS course, combined with ongoing medication and ERP therapy, Mandi's symptoms had improved substantially more than with medication and ERP alone. Her daily ritual time decreased to about forty-five minutes—still present, but no longer dominating her life.

"Deep TMS wasn't a magic cure," Mandi clarified. "I still have OCD. But it gave me enough additional relief that I could finally start living my life instead of just managing symptoms. Combined with the medication and therapy, it was the combination that finally worked for me."

Not everyone needs Deep TMS for OCD treatment—many people respond well to medication and ERP therapy alone. But for those who don't achieve sufficient improvement with first-line treatments, Deep TMS represents an important additional option supported by both controlled research and real-world clinical evidence, including long-term outcome data demonstrating sustained benefits.[18]

THE ROLE OF MEDICATION

After three months on sertraline 150mg daily, Mandi noticed a definite difference. The obsessive thoughts still occurred, but they were less frequent and less distressing. More importantly, she found it easier to resist the compulsions—the anxiety they provoked wasn't quite as overwhelming.

"The medication didn't cure the OCD," Mandi explained. "But it turned down the volume on the obsessions. Instead of the thoughts screaming at me, they were more like background noise. That made doing the ERP exercises much more manageable."

Research shows that combining medication with ERP therapy produces better outcomes than either treatment alone for most people with moderate to severe OCD.[19] The medication helps reduce the intensity of symptoms, making it easier to engage in the challenging work of exposure therapy.

However, medication wasn't without side effects. Mandi experienced some initial nausea, decreased libido, and slight weight gain—common side effects of SSRIs. We adjusted her dose and timing to minimize these effects, and she decided that the improvement in her OCD symptoms was worth the manageable side effects.

"I had to make peace with the fact that treatment isn't perfect," Mandi reflected. "The medication has side effects. The ERP is hard work. The

Deep TMS required daily clinic visits for six weeks. But compared to spending four hours a day trapped in rituals, feeling controlled by my own brain, these are minor inconveniences."

COMMON OCD THEMES

As Mandi progressed in treatment, she learned that her specific obsessions and compulsions fit into common themes seen in OCD. Understanding this helped her feel less alone and recognize that OCD symptoms, while they feel unique and personal, actually follow predictable patterns.[20]

Contamination: Fear of germs, dirt, illness, or being dirty. Compulsions include excessive washing, cleaning, and avoidance of "contaminated" objects or places.

Harm: Intrusive thoughts about causing harm to oneself or others (like Mandi's early fear of hitting someone with her car). Compulsions include checking, seeking reassurance, and avoiding situations where harm could occur.

Symmetry and ordering: Need for things to be perfect, symmetrical, or in exact order. Compulsions include arranging, organizing, and counting until things feel "just right."

Intrusive thoughts: Unwanted thoughts about violence, sex, religion, or other taboo subjects. Compulsions often involve mental rituals like counting, praying, or replacing "bad" thoughts with "good" ones.

Hoarding: Difficulty discarding items due to fear of needing them or losing something important. (This is now considered a separate but related disorder.)

"Learning that other people have similar obsessions was so validating," Mandi said. "I thought my specific fears were bizarre and that I was the only person who worried about these things. Knowing that these are common patterns in OCD helped me externalize the disorder—it wasn't 'me,' it was OCD using common tricks on my brain."

LIFE BEYOND OCD

Eighteen months after beginning treatment, Mandi had made remarkable progress. Her daily ritual time had decreased from four to five hours to approximately thirty minutes. She could leave her house after checking the stove and locks just once. She washed her hands a normal number of times per day. She could tolerate slight imperfections in her environment without experiencing overwhelming anxiety.

"I'm not 'cured,'" Mandi clarified. "I still have obsessive thoughts sometimes, and I still feel urges to check or clean excessively. But now I have tools to manage those urges. I can recognize an OCD thought and choose not to engage with it. Most days, the OCD is background noise rather than the main feature of my life."

Mandi's improvement allowed her to reclaim time and energy for her actual life. She took on new clients at work, knowing she could now complete projects efficiently without getting stuck in rituals. She started dating again, no longer too exhausted or ashamed to let someone into her life. She even adopted a cat—something she had avoided for years due to contamination fears about pet germs.

"The cat was a huge exposure for me," Mandi laughed. "But Dr. Chen encouraged me to do it as a way to practice sitting with uncertainty—I can't control what the cat touches or where she walks. Having her has forced me to be more flexible and accept that some level of mess and unpredictability is normal and okay."

Research on long-term outcomes for OCD shows that with appropriate treatment, approximately 40-50% of people experience significant improvement or remission, while another 30-40% show moderate improvement.[21] Mandi's outcome—substantial improvement with some residual symptoms—represents a typical successful treatment response.

ONGOING MANAGEMENT

Mandi continued to see Dr. Chen monthly for "booster" sessions to maintain her gains and address new situations that triggered OCD symptoms. She also continued taking her medication, having tried to reduce it once with unfortunate results.

"About a year into treatment, I felt so much better that I thought I didn't need the medication anymore," Mandi admitted. "I gradually reduced my dose with my doctor's supervision, but within a few weeks, the obsessive thoughts came back strong. I realized the medication was still helping, even if I didn't notice it day-to-day."

This experience taught Mandi an important lesson about chronic illness management: just because symptoms improve doesn't mean the underlying condition has disappeared. Many people with OCD require long-term medication to maintain their improvement, similar to how people with diabetes need ongoing insulin or people with high blood pressure need ongoing medication.[4]

Mandi also learned to recognize her early warning signs of OCD worsening—increased checking, more elaborate hand-washing, difficulty leaving the house—and to implement immediate interventions. When she noticed these signs, she would increase her ERP practice, reduce stressors where possible, and schedule an extra appointment with Dr. Chen.

"OCD is part of my life, but it doesn't control my life anymore," Mandi reflected. "I've learned to manage it the way someone manages any chronic condition—with ongoing treatment, attention to warning signs, and quick intervention when symptoms worsen. It's not perfect, but it's sustainable."

THE IMPACT OF STIGMA

One of the most challenging aspects of Mandi's journey was dealing with stigma and misunderstanding about OCD. The term "OCD" is often used casually in everyday conversation ("I'm so OCD about my desk being organized!"), which trivializes the genuine suffering of people with the disorder.

"When I finally told some friends about my OCD, several of them said things like, 'Oh, I'm kind of OCD too—I like things neat!'" Mandi recalled. "They didn't understand that what I was describing wasn't about preferences or personality traits. It was about being trapped in a cycle of anxiety and rituals that consumed hours of every day and made me feel like I was losing my mind."

Mandi also encountered healthcare providers who didn't understand OCD. Her previous primary care physician had told her to "just stop worrying so much" and had failed to recognize her symptoms as OCD, despite her washing her hands until they bled and being chronically late to appointments due to checking rituals.

"The misunderstanding and trivialization of OCD is harmful," Mandi emphasized. "It kept me from seeking help for years because I thought everyone experienced intrusive thoughts and that I was just weak for not being able to ignore them. People need to understand that OCD is a serious disorder that requires professional treatment, not just willpower or personality change."

HELPING OTHERS SEEK TREATMENT

Mandi's recovery inspired her to become an advocate for OCD awareness and treatment. She joined the International OCD Foundation (IOCDF) and participated in their advocacy efforts to increase public understanding of the disorder and improve access to evidence-based treatment.

"So many people with OCD suffer in silence for years because they're ashamed or don't realize that treatment exists," Mandi explained. "I want people to know that OCD is treatable. Yes, it's hard work. Yes, it requires confronting your fears. But on the other side of that hard work is freedom from the tyranny of obsessions and compulsions."

Mandi created a blog where she wrote honestly about her experiences with OCD and treatment, including the challenges and setbacks. She received messages from readers all over the world thanking her for helping them understand their own symptoms and encouraging them to seek help.

"If my story helps even one person recognize their OCD and get treatment sooner than I did, then sharing my experience will have been worth it," Mandi said. "No one should have to suffer for fifteen years before getting help, the way I did."

LESSONS FROM MANDI'S JOURNEY

Mandi's story illustrates several crucial points about OCD:

OCD is more than being neat or organized. True OCD involves intrusive, distressing thoughts and time-consuming compulsions that significantly impair functioning. It's a neurobiological disorder, not a personality trait or preference.

Many people suffer in silence for years. Shame, lack of awareness, and misunderstanding about OCD lead many people to hide their symptoms for years or decades before seeking treatment. Early intervention improves outcomes.

ERP therapy is effective but challenging. Exposure and Response Prevention requires deliberately triggering anxiety and resisting compulsions—difficult work that requires courage and persistence. However, it's the most effective treatment for OCD.

Medication helps many people with OCD. SSRIs at higher doses can significantly reduce OCD symptoms, especially when combined with ERP therapy. Many people require long-term medication to maintain improvement.

Deep TMS offers hope for treatment-resistant cases. For people who don't respond adequately to medication and ERP therapy alone, Deep TMS provides an evidence-based option that can produce significant additional improvement with sustained benefits.

Recovery doesn't mean perfection. Most people with OCD who complete treatment still experience some symptoms, but these symptoms no longer control their lives. The goal is management, not elimination of all symptoms.

OCD can improve significantly with treatment. While OCD is a chronic condition, appropriate treatment can lead to dramatic improvements in symptoms and quality of life. Many people go from being severely impaired to living full, productive lives.

Ongoing management is important. OCD symptoms can worsen during stress or if treatment is discontinued. Long-term management strategies help maintain gains and prevent relapse.

A MESSAGE OF HOPE

Mandi's journey from suffering in silence for fifteen years to living a life largely free from OCD's control demonstrates the power of evidence-based treatment. While her path required courage, persistence, and hard work, the results transformed her life.

"If I could go back and tell my seventeen-year-old self something, it would be this: 'What you're experiencing has a name—OCD—and it's treatable,'" Mandi reflected. "I would tell her not to waste fifteen years being ashamed and hiding her symptoms. I would tell her that asking for help isn't weakness, it's wisdom.

"And to anyone reading this who recognizes their own struggles in my story, I want to say: you don't have to keep living this way. OCD can feel overwhelming and permanent, but it's not. With the right treatment—especially ERP therapy and often medication—you can break free from the cycle of obsessions and compulsions. Your life can be about more than managing anxiety and performing rituals.

"Is it easy? No. Is it worth it? Absolutely. The time and energy I've reclaimed, the freedom from constant anxiety, the ability to be present in my life rather than trapped in my head—these are gifts beyond measure. If I can do it after fifteen years of severe symptoms, so can you."

Treatment for OCD is highly effective, with research showing that 60-80% of people who complete a course of ERP therapy experience significant improvement.[1] The key is finding providers trained in evidence-based treatments and committing to the hard work of facing fears and resisting compulsions.

Mandi's story reminds us that even disorders that have persisted for many years and significantly impaired functioning can improve dramatically with appropriate treatment. OCD may be a chronic condition, but it doesn't have to be a life sentence of suffering. With proper help, people with OCD can reclaim their lives and discover that freedom from compulsions is not only possible—it's achievable.

FOOTNOTES

1. Foa, E. B., Liebowitz, M. R., Kozak, M. J., et al. (2005). Randomized, placebo-controlled trial of exposure and ritual prevention, clomipramine, and their combination in the treatment of obsessive-compulsive disorder. *American Journal of Psychiatry, 162*(1), 151-161.# Chapter 7: Mandi's Struggle - Breaking Free from OCD's Grip ↩ ↩[2]

2. Ruscio, A. M., Stein, D. J., Chiu, W. T., & Kessler, R. C. (2010). The epidemiology of obsessive-compulsive disorder in the National Comorbidity Survey Replication. *Molecular Psychiatry, 15*(1), 53-63. ↩

3. American Psychiatric Association. (2013). *Diagnostic and Statistical Manual of Mental Disorders* (5th ed.). Arlington, VA: American Psychiatric Publishing. ↩

4. Geller, D. A., Biederman, J., Jones, J., et al. (1998). Is juvenile obsessive-compulsive disorder a developmental subtype of the disorder? A review of the pediatric literature. *Journal of the American Academy of Child & Adolescent Psychiatry, 37*(4), 420-427. ↩

5. Pinto, A., Mancebo, M. C., Eisen, J. L., Pagano, M. E., & Rasmussen, S. A. (2006). The Brown Longitudinal Obsessive Compulsive Study: clinical features and symptoms of the sample at intake. *Journal of Clinical Psychiatry, 67*(5), 703-711. ↩

6. Saxena, S., Brody, A. L., Schwartz, J. M., & Baxter, L. R. (1998). Neuroimaging and frontal-subcortical circuitry in obsessive-compulsive disorder. *British Journal of Psychiatry, 173*(Suppl 35), 26-37. ↩

7. Soomro, G. M., Altman, D., Rajagopal, S., & Oakley-Browne, M. (2008). Selective serotonin re-uptake inhibitors (SSRIs) versus placebo for obsessive compulsive disorder (OCD). *Cochrane Database of Systematic Reviews, 1*, CD001765. ↩

8. Koran, L. M., Hanna, G. L., Hollander, E., Nestadt, G., & Simpson, H. B. (2007). Practice guideline for the treatment of patients with

obsessive-compulsive disorder. *American Journal of Psychiatry, 164*(7 Suppl), 5-53. ↩

9. Olatunji, B. O., Davis, M. L., Powers, M. B., & Smits, J. A. (2013). Cognitive-behavioral therapy for obsessive-compulsive disorder: a meta-analysis of treatment outcome and moderators. *Journal of Psychiatric Research, 47*(1), 33-41. ↩

10. Simpson, H. B., Foa, E. B., Liebowitz, M. R., et al. (2013). Cognitive-behavioral therapy vs risperidone for augmenting serotonin reuptake inhibitors in obsessive-compulsive disorder: a randomized clinical trial. *JAMA Psychiatry, 70*(11), 1190-1199. ↩

11. Eisen, J. L., Sibrava, N. J., Boisseau, C. L., et al. (2013). Five-year course of obsessive-compulsive disorder: predictors of remission and relapse. *Journal of Clinical Psychiatry, 74*(3), 233-239. ↩

12. Carmi, L., Tendler, A., Bystritsky, A., et al. (2019). Efficacy and safety of deep transcranial magnetic stimulation for obsessive-compulsive disorder: a prospective multicenter randomized double-blind placebo-controlled trial. *American Journal of Psychiatry, 176*(11), 931-938. ↩ ↩[2]

13. Roth, Y., Zangen, A., & Hallett, M. (2002). A coil design for transcranial magnetic stimulation of deep brain regions. *Journal of Clinical Neurophysiology, 19*(4), 361-370. ↩ ↩[2]

14. Dunlop, K., Woodside, B., Lam, E., et al. (2015). Increases in frontostriatal connectivity are associated with response to dorsomedial repetitive transcranial magnetic stimulation in obsessive-compulsive disorder. *Brain Stimulation, 9*(6), 890-896. ↩

15. Carmi, L., Tendler, A., Bystritsky, A., et al. (2019). Efficacy and safety of deep transcranial magnetic stimulation for obsessive-compulsive disorder: a prospective multicenter randomized double-blind placebo-controlled trial. *American Journal of Psychiatry, 176*(11), 931-938. ↩

16. Roth, Y., Tendler, A., Arikan, M. K., Vidrine, R., Kent, D., Muir, O., MacMillan, C., Casuto, L., Grammer, G., Sauve, W., Tolin, K., Harvey, S., Borst, M., Rifkin, R., Sheth, M., Cornejo, B., Rodriguez, R., Shakir, S., Porter, T., Kim, D., Peterson, B., Swofford, J., Roe, B., Sinclair, R., Harmelech, T., & Zangen, A. (2021). Real-world efficacy of deep TMS for obsessive-compulsive disorder: Post-marketing data collected from twenty-two clinical sites. *Journal of Psychiatric Research, 137*, 667-672. ↩

17. Roth, Y., Zangen, A., & Hallett, M. (2002). A coil design for transcranial magnetic stimulation of deep brain regions. *Journal of Clinical Neurophysiology, 19*(4), 361-370. ↩

18. Trevizol, A. P., Shiozawa, P., Cook, I. A., et al. (2016). Transcranial magnetic stimulation for obsessive-compulsive disorder: an updated systematic review and meta-analysis. *Journal of ECT, 32*(4), 262-266. ↩

19. Skoog, G., & Skoog, I. (1999). A 40-year follow-up of patients with obsessive-compulsive disorder. *Archives of General Psychiatry, 56*(2), 121-127. ↩

20. Fineberg, N. A., Brown, A., Reghunandanan, S., & Pampaloni, I. (2012). Evidence-based pharmacotherapy of obsessive-compulsive disorder. *International Journal of Neuropsychopharmacology, 15*(8), 1173-1191. ↩

21. Abramowitz, J. S. (1997). Effectiveness of psychological and pharmacological treatments for obsessive-compulsive disorder: a quantitative review. *Journal of Consulting and Clinical Psychology, 65*(1), 44-52. ↩

CHAPTER 8
RACHEL'S STORM – NAVIGATING BORDERLINE PERSONALITY DISORDER

Rachel was 26 when she first came to my office, though it wasn't the first time she had sought psychiatric help. Over the previous eight years, she had seen five different therapists, been hospitalized three times for suicidal gestures, and cycled through various medications with little sustained improvement. Her arms bore the faint white scars of years of self-harm, hidden beneath long sleeves even in summer.

"I don't know why I'm here," she said during our first session. "Nothing ever helps. Every therapist eventually gives up on me. I'm probably just wasting your time too."

This dismissive opening belied the desperation underneath—a desperation born from years of intense emotional pain, turbulent relationships, and a persistent feeling of emptiness. Rachel's story illustrates the complex reality of Borderline Personality Disorder (BPD), one of the most misunderstood and stigmatized mental health conditions.

UNDERSTANDING BORDERLINE PERSONALITY DISORDER

Borderline Personality Disorder affects approximately 1.4% of the adult population, though rates are higher in clinical settings.[1] The disorder is characterized by a pervasive pattern of instability in relationships, self-image, and emotions, along with marked impulsivity.

The DSM-5 identifies nine criteria for BPD, with at least five required for diagnosis:[2]

Frantic efforts to avoid real or imagined abandonment
Pattern of unstable and intense interpersonal relationships
Identity disturbance: markedly unstable self-image
Impulsivity in at least two self-damaging areas
Recurrent suicidal behavior, gestures, or self-harm
Affective instability and mood reactivity
Chronic feelings of emptiness
Inappropriate, intense anger or difficulty controlling anger
Transient, stress-related paranoid ideation or dissociative symptoms
Rachel met seven of these criteria. Understanding the diagnosis was just the beginning of a long treatment journey.

THE ROOTS OF RACHEL'S PAIN

Rachel's childhood was marked by trauma and instability. Her father struggled with alcoholism and was verbally abusive when drunk, alternating between emotional unavailability and explosive anger. Her mother, overwhelmed and depressed, was inconsistently available.

"I never knew which version of my parents I was going to get," Rachel recalled. "I learned early that people I loved could disappear at any moment, even when they were standing right in front of me."

This early environment of invalidation and unpredictability is common in BPD histories.[3] Children in chaotic or emotionally invalidating environments often don't learn healthy ways to identify, express, or regulate their emotions. They develop intense fear of abandonment and difficulty trusting others.

Rachel's self-harm began at age 14, after her first serious relationship ended. "The emotional pain was so intense that cutting myself was the only thing that brought relief," she explained. "The physical pain was something I could control."

THE PATTERN OF INSTABILITY

By her mid-twenties, a clear pattern had emerged. Rachel would meet someone new and quickly idealize them—they were perfect, wonderful, the answer to all her problems. She would become intensely attached, overwhelming the other person with her neediness.

"When I met someone I really connected with, they became my whole world," Rachel explained. "I would text them constantly, want to spend all my time with them."

But inevitably, something would trigger her. The person would be unavailable when Rachel needed them or make a comment she perceived as critical. Her idealization would flip instantly to devaluation.

"I would go from thinking someone was the best person in the world to hating them in an instant," Rachel admitted. "And both feelings were completely real to me in the moment."

This splitting—seeing people as all good or all bad—is a hallmark of BPD.[4] Her romantic relationships typically lasted a few months and followed a predictable pattern: intense idealization, jealousy and fear of abandonment, angry outbursts or desperate attempts to prevent the partner from leaving, and ultimately the relationship ending.

THE EMOTIONAL ROLLER COASTER

Rachel's emotional instability was particularly distressing. Her moods could shift rapidly and intensely in response to seemingly small triggers.

An unanswered text could send her into despair. A perceived slight could trigger intense rage.

"My emotions felt like a roller coaster that never stopped," Rachel described. "I would wake up feeling okay, but by lunchtime I'd be in despair, by dinner furious, and by bedtime numb and empty."

This emotional dysregulation differs from bipolar disorder.[5] In BPD, mood changes are typically reactive to interpersonal events and last hours rather than days. Rachel also struggled with chronic emptiness—a disturbing sense that something essential was missing inside her.

"It's not sadness," she explained. "It's more like being hollow, like there's a void inside me that nothing can fill."

This emptiness drove much of Rachel's impulsive behavior: binge eating, reckless spending, risky sexual behavior, substance use—all attempts to feel something, to fill the void.

THE FUNCTION OF SELF-HARM

Rachel's self-harm was one of her most concerning symptoms. She cut her arms and thighs with razors, burned herself with cigarettes, and occasionally hit herself when overwhelmed.

"People think self-harm is a suicide attempt, but it's not—at least not for me," Rachel explained. "When I'm feeling overwhelming emotional pain, cutting releases some of that pressure. The physical pain distracts from the emotional pain."

Research shows that self-harm in BPD often serves multiple functions: emotion regulation, self-punishment, communication of distress, and generation of feeling when numb.[6] Rachel also engaged in suicidal gestures—non-lethal overdoses after relationship crises.

"I didn't really want to die," Rachel admitted. "But I wanted the pain to stop, and I wanted people to understand how much I was hurting."

People with BPD are at significant risk for completed suicide, with rates approximately 50 times higher than the general population.[7] Every self-harm behavior must be taken seriously.

THE STRUGGLE WITH IDENTITY

Rachel struggled with a profound sense of not knowing who she was. Her values, goals, and personality seemed to shift depending on whom she was with.

"I'm like a chameleon," Rachel said. "I don't know what I actually like when I'm alone. I don't know who the real Rachel is."

This identity disturbance is a core feature of BPD.[8] Rachel had changed college majors four times before dropping out and held jobs in completely unrelated fields. This lack of stable identity made it difficult to set long-term goals.

DISCOVERING DIALECTICAL BEHAVIOR THERAPY

I explained to Rachel that her previous treatment failures didn't mean she was untreatable—she hadn't yet received the right kind of treatment. Dialectical Behavior Therapy (DBT), developed specifically for BPD by psychologist Marsha Linehan, was a viable option. [9]

"DBT is based on understanding that people with BPD have difficulties regulating emotions due to biological vulnerability combined with invalidating environments," I explained. "DBT teaches specific skills for managing emotions, tolerating distress, improving relationships, and developing mindfulness."

DBT involves individual therapy, skills training groups, phone coaching for crises, and a consultation team for therapists. Rachel was skeptical—she had tried therapy before. But DBT's dialectical approach—balancing acceptance and change—is what makes it effective.[10]

LEARNING NEW SKILLS

Rachel began weekly DBT skills group. The group taught four skill modules:

Mindfulness: Learning to be present without judgment. "I started to notice that most of my suffering came from thoughts about the past or future, not what was actually happening now," Rachel said.

Distress Tolerance: Surviving crises without making them worse. Rachel learned alternatives to cutting—holding ice cubes, taking cold showers, intense exercise. "The distress tolerance skills gave me options," Rachel explained.

Emotion Regulation: Understanding emotions and changing unwanted responses. Rachel learned that emotions naturally rise and fall. "I always thought if I started feeling angry, it would keep getting worse forever unless I did something drastic," she said.

Interpersonal Effectiveness: Asking for needs, saying no, managing conflicts. "I was either completely passive or aggressive," Rachel reflected. "I didn't know there was a middle ground."

THE HARD WORK OF CHANGE

Progress was slow. Rachel would have weeks of practicing skills and feeling stable, then a crisis would trigger a spiral. In her first three months of DBT, Rachel cut herself 23 times. In months four through six, it was 12 times. By months seven through nine, it was 5 times.

"My emotions told me nothing was changing, but the data showed I was using healthier coping strategies more often," Rachel explained.

The phone coaching proved valuable. When in crisis, Rachel could call for help using skills. "Knowing I could reach out between sessions changed everything," she said.

A major focus was examining relationship patterns. Rachel discovered her fear of abandonment led to behaviors that pushed people away—a self-fulfilling prophecy.

"When I sensed distance, I would panic and text constantly, get angry, make threats," Rachel said. "Of course that drove them away. I was creating the very thing I feared."

She learned to check the facts, tolerate uncertainty, and communicate needs more effectively. "When my boyfriend didn't text back for three hours, my new pattern was to notice my anxiety, use skills, and send one message saying I felt anxious. That actually worked better."

ADDRESSING TRAUMA

As Rachel became more stable, we addressed childhood trauma. Many people with BPD have histories of abuse, neglect, or invalidation.[11] Processing these experiences is important for recovery.

"I realized I learned that relationships were dangerous," Rachel said. "I was applying childhood survival strategies to adult relationships where they didn't fit."

Processing this trauma helped Rachel develop compassion for herself. She began seeing her BPD symptoms not as defects, but as understandable responses to difficult experiences combined with biological vulnerability.

TWO YEARS INTO TREATMENT

After two years of consistent DBT, Rachel's life looked dramatically different. She hadn't self-harmed for nine months. She had maintained a job for over a year. She was in a healthier, more stable romantic relationship.

"I still have BPD," Rachel clarified. "I still feel emotions intensely. But now I have tools to manage those experiences without destroying my life."

Her hospitalizations dropped from 2-3 per year to zero in 18 months. Her ER visits for self-harm went from monthly to none. Studies show that comprehensive DBT significantly reduces self-harm, suicidal behavior, and hospitalizations.[12]

BUILDING A LIFE WORTH LIVING

A central DBT concept is building a "life worth living." For Rachel, this meant pursuing values and goals beyond managing BPD. She returned to college for a degree in social work.

"I want to help other people who struggle the way I have," she explained. "My experience could make me a better therapist."

Rachel developed healthier friendships and joined a DBT alumni group. She discovered that her emotional sensitivity allowed for intense joy, deep empathy, and creative expression. She started painting.

"My emotional intensity isn't all bad," Rachel reflected. "Once I learned to manage the pain, I could appreciate the depth of feeling as a gift."

LONG-TERM OUTLOOK

After five years of treatment, Rachel completed her degree and works as a case manager at a community mental health center. She continues maintenance DBT sessions and skills practice. Her self-harm has been absent for over two years. She's been in a stable relationship for 18 months.

"I'm not cured," Rachel emphasizes. "BPD is still part of who I am. But those experiences don't control my life anymore."

Research shows that with proper treatment, the majority of people with BPD show significant improvement over time.[13] While some symptoms may persist, functioning typically improves dramatically.

LESSONS FROM RACHEL'S JOURNEY

Rachel's story illustrates several crucial points about BPD:

BPD is rooted in biology and environment. The combination of emotional sensitivity and invalidating early experiences creates BPD patterns. It's not a choice or character flaw.

Previous treatment failures don't predict future outcomes. Many people try multiple treatments before finding DBT. Generic therapy failures don't mean the person is untreatable.

Self-harm serves functions. Understanding why people engage in these behaviors is crucial. These actions regulate emotions or communicate distress.

Specialized therapy is essential. DBT and other evidence-based treatments specifically designed for BPD are far more effective than generic approaches.

Improvement takes time. Rachel spent five years in treatment to achieve her current functioning. BPD treatment requires patience and persistence.

Recovery doesn't mean perfection. Rachel still has BPD symptoms, but they no longer dominate her life. The goal is effective management.

Emotional intensity can be channeled positively. The same sensitivity that causes pain enables deep empathy, creativity, and passion when managed.

Relationships can improve dramatically. With skills training, people with BPD can develop healthier relationship patterns.

A MESSAGE OF HOPE

Rachel's transformation demonstrates that BPD, despite its severity, is treatable. The path requires finding the right treatment, committing to intensive therapy, and developing skills to manage intense emotions.

"If I could tell someone newly diagnosed with BPD one thing, it would be: you're not hopeless," Rachel said. "With the right treatment and enough time, you can build a life that feels worth living.

"Will it be easy? No. DBT was the hardest thing I've ever done. But it was worth it. I have a real life now with work I care about, relationships that sustain me, and a future I'm excited about.

"You don't have to be perfect. You just have to learn to manage symptoms well enough that they don't destroy everything you care about. That's possible. I'm living proof."

For families and loved ones: "Don't give up on us. We're not manipulating you. We're struggling with pain you can't see. Be patient. Recovery takes time, but it does happen."

Borderline Personality Disorder carries significant stigma, even within mental health. Some clinicians refuse to treat people with BPD, viewing them as manipulative or treatment-resistant. This stigma compounds suffering.

Rachel's story challenges these stereotypes. With appropriate treatment, people with BPD can develop insight, learn skills, change patterns, and build meaningful lives. The development of DBT represents a major advance in psychiatry.

Rachel's journey from chaos to stability demonstrates that recovery from BPD is achievable with proper treatment, committed effort, and time. Her story offers hope to people struggling with this challenging disorder and to families supporting them.

FOOTNOTES

1. Grant, B. F., Chou, S. P., Goldstein, R. B., et al. (2008). Prevalence, correlates, disability, and comorbidity of DSM-IV borderline personality disorder. *Journal of Clinical Psychiatry, 69*(4), 533-545. ↩

2. American Psychiatric Association. (2013). *Diagnostic and Statistical Manual of Mental Disorders* (5th ed.). Arlington, VA: American Psychiatric Publishing. ↩

3. Crowell, S. E., Beauchaine, T. P., & Linehan, M. M. (2009). A biosocial developmental model of borderline personality. *Psychological Bulletin, 135*(3), 495-510. ↩

4. Veen, G., & Arntz, A. (2000). Multidimensional dichotomous thinking characterizes borderline personality disorder. *Cognitive Therapy and Research, 24*(1), 23-45. ↩

5. Henry, C., Mitropoulou, V., New, A. S., et al. (2001). Affective instability and impulsivity in borderline personality and bipolar II disorders. *Journal of Psychiatric Research, 35*(6), 307-312. ↩

6. Klonsky, E. D. (2007). The functions of deliberate self-injury. *Clinical Psychology Review, 27*(2), 226-239. ↩

7. Paris, J., & Zweig-Frank, H. (2001). A 27-year follow-up of patients with borderline personality disorder. *Comprehensive Psychiatry, 42*(6), 482-487. ↩

8. Wilkinson-Ryan, T., & Westen, D. (2000). Identity disturbance in borderline personality disorder. *American Journal of Psychiatry, 157*(4), 528-541. ↩

9. Linehan, M. M., Armstrong, H. E., Suarez, A., Allmon, D., & Heard, H. L. (1991). Cognitive-behavioral treatment of chronically parasuicidal borderline patients. *Archives of General Psychiatry, 48*(12), 1060-1064. ↩

10. Lynch, T. R., Chapman, A. L., Rosenthal, M. Z., Kuo, J. R., & Linehan, M. M. (2006). Mechanisms of change in dialectical behavior therapy. *Journal of Clinical Psychology, 62*(4), 459-480. ↩

11. Ball, J. S., & Links, P. S. (2009). Borderline personality disorder and childhood trauma. *Current Psychiatry Reports, 11*(1), 63-68. ↩

12. Linehan, M. M., Comtois, K. A., Murray, A. M., et al. (2006). Two-year randomized controlled trial of dialectical behavior therapy vs therapy by experts for suicidal behaviors and borderline personality disorder. *Archives of General Psychiatry, 63*(7), 757-766. ↩

13. Zanarini, M. C., Frankenburg, F. R., Reich, D. B., & Fitzmaurice, G. (2012). Attainment and stability of sustained symptomatic remission and recovery among patients with borderline personality disorder. *American Journal of Psychiatry, 169*(5), 476-483. ↩

PART III

HOPE, TREATMENT, AND MOVING FORWARD

CHAPTER 9
THE SCIENCE OF TREATMENT - WHAT WORKS AND WHY

After walking alongside Sarah through her depression, Marcus through his bipolar journey, David's experience with schizophrenia, Mandi's struggle with OCD, Rachel's navigation of borderline personality disorder, and James' journey with Schizoaffective Disorder you've seen the profound impact that mental health conditions can have on every aspect of a person's life. But you've also witnessed something equally important: the remarkable capacity for recovery and healing when people receive appropriate treatment.

The stories in this book aren't exceptions—they represent the norm for what's possible when mental health conditions are properly understood and treated. The key phrase here is "properly treated," because not all mental health interventions are created equal. In this chapter, we'll explore the science behind what works in mental health treatment and why these evidence-based approaches are so effective.

THE EVIDENCE-BASED TREATMENT REVOLUTION

Mental health treatment has undergone a revolution over the past several decades. Gone are the days when treatment decisions were based primarily on theoretical orientations or personal preferences. Today's most effective treatments are backed by rigorous scientific research demonstrating their safety and efficacy.

Evidence-based treatment means that interventions have been tested through controlled studies, their effects have been measured objectively, and their benefits have been replicated across different populations and settings.[1] This scientific approach has led to remarkable improvements in outcomes for virtually every mental health condition.

When I started practicing psychiatry decades ago, our treatment options were much more limited. Today, we have dozens of proven interventions for conditions that once carried poor prognoses. The difference is that we now know not just what works, but how and why it works.

BIOLOGICAL TREATMENTS: MEDICATIONS AND BEYOND

The biological basis of mental illness we explored in Chapter 1 means that many conditions benefit significantly from interventions that target brain chemistry and function. These treatments work by correcting the neurochemical imbalances and neural dysfunction that underlie mental health symptoms.

PSYCHOPHARMACOLOGY: THE MEDICATION REVOLUTION

Modern psychiatric medications are safer, more effective, and better tolerated than ever before. The development of selective serotonin reuptake inhibitors (SSRIs) in the 1980s marked a turning point in depression treatment, providing effective relief with fewer side effects than older antidepressants.[2]

Today's medication arsenal includes multiple classes of drugs targeting different neurotransmitter systems:

Antidepressants work by increasing availability of neurotransmitters like serotonin, norepinephrine, and dopamine. Response rates for depression range from 60-70% when medications are properly matched to individual patients and given adequate trials.[3]

Mood stabilizers like lithium and anticonvulsants (Depakote, Lamictal, Tegretol, Trileptal) help regulate the extreme mood swings characteristic of bipolar disorder. Lithium, in particular, has been shown to reduce suicide risk by up to 80% in people with bipolar disorder.[4]

Antipsychotic medications target dopamine receptors to reduce hallucinations, delusions, and disordered thinking in conditions like schizophrenia. Newer "atypical" antipsychotics have fewer neurological side effects while maintaining efficacy.[5]

Anti-anxiety medications provide rapid relief for severe anxiety symptoms, though they're typically used short-term due to dependence potential.

The key to successful medication treatment is precision matching. We now understand that people with the same diagnosis may have different underlying biological profiles, requiring different medication approaches. Pharmacogenetic testing can help predict how individuals will respond to certain drugs.[6]

TRANSCRANIAL MAGNETIC STIMULATION (TMS): TARGETED BRAIN STIMULATION

TMS represents one of the most exciting developments in biological psychiatry. This non-invasive procedure uses magnetic fields to stimulate specific brain regions involved in mood regulation. For treatment-resistant depression, TMS shows response rates of 50-60%, with benefits often lasting six months to several years.[7]

TMS was a game-changer for patients who hadn't responded to multiple medication trials. It provides an option for people who had begun to lose hope, and the lack of systemic side effects makes it particularly appealing. As we discussed in Sarah's chapter, TMS offers durability—the only biological treatment where benefits can persist long after treatment ends.

TMS is now being studied for other conditions including anxiety disorders, PTSD, and obsessive-compulsive disorder, with promising preliminary results. Deep TMS (BrainsWay), which we explored in Mandi's chapter, has shown particular promise for treatment-resistant OCD.[8]

Electroconvulsive Therapy (ECT): Still the Gold Standard for Severe Depression

Despite its historical stigma, ECT remains one of the most effective treatments for severe depression, with response rates of 80-90%.[9] Modern ECT is performed under anesthesia with muscle relaxants, making it much safer and more comfortable than historical procedures.

ECT literally saves lives. For people with severe, life-threatening depression who haven't responded to other treatments, ECT can provide rapid, dramatic improvement. The temporary memory effects are usually acceptable given the profound benefits.

Ketamine Therapy: Rapid-Acting Relief

Ketamine represents a breakthrough in understanding depression neurobiology. Unlike traditional antidepressants that work on monoamine neurotransmitter levels, ketamine targets the brain's glutamate system, producing rapid antidepressant effects—sometimes within hours rather than weeks.[10]

Esketamine (Spravato), a nasal spray form of ketamine, is now FDA-approved for treatment-resistant depression and provides hope for people who haven't responded to traditional medications. However, as discussed in Sarah's chapter, ketamine's effects are often temporary, requiring ongoing treatments to maintain benefits.

Psychological Treatments: The Power of Therapy

While biological treatments target the physical aspects of mental illness, psychological therapies address the cognitive, emotional, and behavioral components. The most effective therapies are based on scientific understanding of how thoughts, feelings, and behaviors interact to maintain mental health problems.

Cognitive-Behavioral Therapy (CBT): The Most Studied Approach

CBT is based on the principle that our thoughts, feelings, and behaviors are interconnected, and that changing one component can positively affect the others. CBT has been extensively studied and proven effective for depression, anxiety disorders, PTSD, eating disorders, and many other conditions.[11]

CBT gives people practical tools for managing their symptoms. Rather than just talking about problems, we teach specific skills for identifying and changing unhelpful thought patterns and behaviors. Sarah's experience with CBT helped her recognize and challenge the negative thinking patterns that maintained her depression.

CBT's effectiveness comes from its focus on:
Identifying and challenging distorted thinking patterns
Behavioral activation and exposure to feared situations
Problem-solving skills training
Relapse prevention strategies

Meta-analyses show that CBT is as effective as antidepressant medication for moderate depression, with lower relapse rates when treatment ends.[12]

Dialectical Behavior Therapy (DBT): Specialized Skills for Emotional Regulation

DBT was developed specifically for borderline personality disorder but has proven effective for any condition involving emotional dysregulation. The therapy teaches four core skill sets: mindfulness, emotional regulation, distress tolerance, and interpersonal effectiveness.[13]

As Rachel discovered in her treatment, DBT provides specific tools for managing intense emotions without destroying relationships or engaging in self-harm. The skills become automatic with practice, transforming how people respond to emotional challenges.

Research shows that DBT significantly reduces self-harm behaviors, hospitalizations, and relationship chaos while improving overall functioning and quality of life.[14]

Exposure and Response Prevention (ERP): The Gold Standard for OCD

ERP is the most effective psychological treatment for OCD, with success rates of 60-80%.[15] As Mandi experienced, ERP involves deliberately triggering obsessive thoughts while resisting compulsive behaviors, allowing the brain to learn that anxiety decreases naturally without rituals.

While challenging, ERP produces lasting changes in how the brain processes obsessive thoughts and provides tools that continue working long after therapy ends.

Trauma-Focused Therapies: Healing from the Past

For conditions rooted in traumatic experiences, specialized trauma therapies have proven remarkably effective:[16]

Eye Movement Desensitization and Reprocessing (EMDR) uses bilateral stimulation to help process traumatic memories, reducing their emotional impact.

Prolonged Exposure therapy gradually helps people confront trauma-related memories and situations they've been avoiding.

Cognitive Processing Therapy addresses the thoughts and beliefs that develop after trauma.

These therapies work by helping the brain process traumatic experiences in a healthier way. Instead of avoiding trauma memories, we help people integrate them in a way that reduces their ongoing impact.

Acceptance and Commitment Therapy (ACT): Psychological Flexibility

ACT focuses on helping people develop psychological flexibility—the ability to stay present with experiences while acting in accordance with personal values. Rather than trying to eliminate difficult thoughts and feelings, ACT teaches acceptance and commitment to meaningful action.[17]

ACT is particularly helpful for people who struggle with accepting their mental health conditions. It teaches that having difficult thoughts and feelings is part of being human, and that we can live meaningful lives even when uncomfortable experiences persist.

Combining Treatments: The Power of Integration

For many mental health conditions, combining biological and psychological treatments produces better outcomes than either approach alone. Sarah's recovery involved both medication and therapy. Marcus benefited from mood stabilizers plus therapy focused on recognizing mood episode warning signs. Mandi's OCD improved most when medication, ERP therapy, and Deep TMS were combined.

Research consistently shows that integrated treatment approaches produce:[18]

Higher response rates
Lower relapse rates
Better overall functioning
Greater treatment satisfaction
Improved quality of life

The key is tailoring treatment combinations to individual needs—what I call "custom work." No single approach works for everyone, which is why having multiple evidence-based options is so important.

Lifestyle Interventions: The Foundation of Mental Health

Beyond formal treatments, lifestyle factors play crucial roles in mental health and recovery. These aren't "alternative" treatments but rather essential foundations that support all other interventions.

Exercise: Moving for Mental Health

Regular physical activity has proven antidepressant and anxiolytic effects comparable to medication for mild to moderate conditions.[19] Exercise promotes neuroplasticity, reduces inflammation, regulates stress hormones, and improves sleep—all mechanisms that support mental health.

The prescription is simple: 30 minutes of moderate exercise most days of the week. Walking, swimming, cycling, dancing—any activity that gets your heart rate up provides benefits.

Sleep: The Brain's Reset Button

Sleep disturbances both cause and result from mental health problems. Prioritizing good sleep hygiene—consistent sleep schedules, dark and cool sleeping environments, limiting screen time before bed—supports every aspect of mental health treatment.[20]

Many of our patients, including Sarah and Marcus, found that improving sleep quality was one of the most impactful changes they made.

Nutrition: Feeding the Brain

Emerging research shows that diet affects mental health through multiple pathways including inflammation, gut microbiome, and neurotransmitter production. Mediterranean-style diets rich in vegetables, fruits, whole grains, fish, and healthy fats show particular promise for supporting mental health.[21]

While nutrition alone rarely treats mental illness, poor nutrition can undermine other treatments, while good nutrition supports recovery.

Social Connection: The Power of Relationships

Humans are inherently social creatures, and strong social connections protect against mental illness while promoting recovery. Loneliness and social isolation, conversely, are significant risk factors for poor mental health outcomes.[22]

Building and maintaining meaningful relationships—whether with family, friends, support groups, or community organizations—should be considered a core component of mental health treatment.

THE ROLE OF TECHNOLOGY IN MODERN TREATMENT

Technology is transforming mental health care delivery and accessibility:

Teletherapy allows people to access specialized treatment regardless of geographic location. Research shows that teletherapy is as effective as in-person treatment for many conditions.[23]

Smartphone apps help people track symptoms, practice skills, and access support between therapy sessions.

Virtual reality is being used for exposure therapy for phobias, PTSD, and anxiety disorders.

AI and machine learning are improving diagnostic accuracy and treatment matching.

These technological advances are making evidence-based treatment more accessible to people who previously faced barriers to care.

MEASURING TREATMENT SUCCESS

Modern mental health treatment emphasizes measurement-based care—regularly assessing symptoms and functioning to guide treatment decisions. This approach improves outcomes by:[24]

Identifying treatments that aren't working quickly
Allowing for timely adjustments to treatment plans
Providing objective feedback on progress
Increasing patient engagement in treatment

Tools like depression rating scales, anxiety inventories, and functioning assessments help track progress and optimize treatment approaches.

THE FUTURE OF MENTAL HEALTH TREATMENT

The field continues to evolve rapidly with exciting developments on the horizon:

Precision psychiatry using genetic, neuroimaging, and biomarker data to match individuals with optimal treatments

Novel drug targets including psychedelics showing promise for treatment-resistant conditions

Neurostimulation advances with more targeted and effective brain stimulation techniques

Prevention focus with early intervention programs reducing incidence of serious mental illness

Global mental health initiatives improving access to evidence-based treatment worldwide

These advances mean that the future holds even greater promise for people facing mental health challenges.

A MESSAGE ABOUT TREATMENT

The most important message about mental health treatment is this: effective help exists. The stories in this book demonstrate that with proper diagnosis, evidence-based treatment, and appropriate support, recovery is not just possible—it's probable.

Treatment works. The science is clear, the evidence is compelling, and the outcomes speak for themselves. Whether through medication, therapy, brain stimulation, lifestyle changes, or—most often—combinations of these approaches, people can and do recover from even severe mental health conditions.

The key is seeking help, engaging with evidence-based treatments, and persisting through the challenges that treatment sometimes involves.

Recovery takes time, effort, and patience. But the destination—a life no longer controlled by mental illness—is worth the journey.

As we've seen through Sarah's, Marcus's, David's, Mandi's, James' and Rachel's stories, proper treatment doesn't just reduce symptoms. It restores hope, rebuilds relationships, enables pursuit of goals, and allows people to live the lives they choose rather than lives dictated by mental illness.

That's the promise of evidence-based mental health treatment. That's what proper care can achieve. And that's why understanding what works—and why it works—is so crucial for anyone touched by mental illness.

FOOTNOTES

1. Chambless, D. L., & Hollon, S. D. (1998). Defining empirically supported therapies. *Journal of Consulting and Clinical Psychology, 66*(1), 7-18. ↩

2. Wong, D. T., Bymaster, F. P., & Engleman, E. A. (1995). Prozac (fluoxetine, Lilly 110140), the first selective serotonin uptake inhibitor and an antidepressant drug. *Life Sciences, 57*(5), 411-441. ↩

3. Rush, A. J., Trivedi, M. H., Wisniewski, S. R., et al. (2006). Acute and longer-term outcomes in depressed outpatients requiring one or several treatment steps: a STAR*D report. *American Journal of Psychiatry, 163*(11), 1905-1917. ↩

4. Cipriani, A., Hawton, K., Stockton, S., & Geddes, J. R. (2013). Lithium in the prevention of suicide in mood disorders: updated systematic review and meta-analysis. *BMJ, 346*, f3646. ↩

5. Leucht, S., Corves, C., Arbter, D., Engel, R. R., Li, C., & Davis, J. M. (2009). Second-generation versus first-generation antipsychotic drugs for schizophrenia: a meta-analysis. *The Lancet, 373*(9657), 31-41. ↩

6. Bousman, C. A., & Dunlop, B. W. (2018). Genotype, phenotype, and medication recommendation for depressive disorders: a systematic review. *Molecular Psychiatry, 23*(7), 1633-1644. ↩

7. Carpenter, L. L., Janicak, P. G., Aaronson, S. T., et al. (2012). Transcranial magnetic stimulation (TMS) for major depression: a multisite, naturalistic, observational study of acute treatment outcomes in clinical practice. *Depression and Anxiety, 29*(7), 587-596. ↩

8. Carmi, L., Tendler, A., Bystritsky, A., et al. (2019). Efficacy and safety of deep transcranial magnetic stimulation for obsessive-compulsive disorder: a prospective multicenter randomized double-blind placebo-controlled trial. *American Journal of Psychiatry, 176*(11), 931-938. ↩

9. UK ECT Review Group. (2003). Efficacy and safety of electroconvulsive therapy in depressive disorders: a systematic review and meta-analysis. *The Lancet, 361*(9360), 799-808. ↩

10. Berman, R. M., Cappiello, A., Anand, A., et al. (2000). Antidepressant effects of ketamine in depressed patients. *Biological Psychiatry, 47*(4), 351-354. ↩

11. Hofmann, S. G., Asnaani, A., Vonk, I. J., Sawyer, A. T., & Fang, A. (2012). The efficacy of cognitive behavioral therapy: a review of meta-analyses. *Cognitive Therapy and Research, 36*(5), 427-440. ↩

12. Hollon, S. D., Stewart, M. O., & Strunk, D. (2006). Enduring effects for cognitive behavior therapy in the treatment of depression and anxiety. *Annual Review of Psychology, 57*, 285-315. ↩

13. Linehan, M. M., Armstrong, H. E., Suarez, A., Allmon, D., & Heard, H. L. (1991). Cognitive-behavioral treatment of chronically parasuicidal borderline patients. *Archives of General Psychiatry, 48*(12), 1060-1064. ↩

14. Linehan, M. M., Comtois, K. A., Murray, A. M., et al. (2006). Two-year randomized controlled trial and follow-up of dialectical behavior therapy vs therapy by experts for suicidal behaviors and borderline personality disorder. *Archives of General Psychiatry, 63*(7), 757-766. ↩

15. Olatunji, B. O., Davis, M. L., Powers, M. B., & Smits, J. A. (2013). Cognitive-behavioral therapy for obsessive-compulsive disorder: a meta-analysis of treatment outcome and moderators. *Journal of Psychiatric Research, 47*(1), 33-41. ↩

16. Cusack, K., Jonas, D. E., Forneris, C. A., et al. (2016). Psychological treatments for adults with posttraumatic stress disorder: a systematic review and meta-analysis. *Clinical Psychology Review, 43*, 128-141. ↩

17. A-Tjak, J. G., Davis, M. L., Morina, N., et al. (2015). A meta-analysis of the efficacy of acceptance and commitment therapy for clinically relevant mental and physical health problems. *Psychotherapy and Psychosomatics, 84*(1), 30-36. ↩

18. Cuijpers, P., Dekker, J., Hollon, S. D., & Andersson, G. (2009). Adding psychotherapy to pharmacotherapy in the treatment of depressive disorders in adults: a meta-analysis. *Journal of Clinical Psychiatry, 70*(9), 1219-1229. ↩

19. Schuch, F. B., Vancampfort, D., Richards, J., Rosenbaum, S., Ward, P. B., & Stubbs, B. (2016). Exercise as a treatment for depression: a meta-analysis. *Journal of Affective Disorders, 202*, 67-86. ↩

20. Baglioni, C., Nanovska, S., Regen, W., et al. (2016). Sleep and mental disorders: a meta-analysis of polysomnographic research. *Psychological Bulletin, 142*(9), 969-990. ↩

21. Lai, J. S., Hiles, S., Bisquera, A., Hure, A. J., McEvoy, M., & Attia, J. (2014). A systematic review and meta-analysis of dietary patterns and depression in community-dwelling adults. *American Journal of Clinical Nutrition, 99*(1), 181-197. ↩

22. Holt-Lunstad, J., Smith, T. B., Baker, M., Harris, T., & Stephenson, D. (2015). Loneliness and social isolation as risk factors for mortality: a meta-analytic review. *Perspectives on Psychological Science, 10*(2), 227-237. ↩

23. Hilty, D. M., Ferrer, D. C., Parish, M. B., Johnston, B., Callahan, E. J., & Yellowlees, P. M. (2013). The effectiveness of telemental health: a 2013 review. *Telemedicine and e-Health, 19*(6), 444-454. ↩

24. Scott, K., & Lewis, C. C. (2015). Using measurement-based care to enhance any treatment. *Cognitive and Behavioral Practice, 22*(1), 49-59. ↩

CHAPTER 10
THE POWER OF FAMILY AND SUPPORT SYSTEMS

When David first started hearing voices during college, his parents felt a mixture of fear, confusion, and helplessness. Like many families confronting mental illness for the first time, they didn't know what to say, how to help, or even how to understand what their son was experiencing. Their journey from bewildered observers to educated advocates illustrates the profound impact that families and support systems can have on mental health recovery.

"Looking back, I realize we made every mistake in the book during David's first months of illness," his mother admitted during our family therapy session. "We tried to reason away his delusions, argued with him about what was real, and desperately searched for someone or something to blame. It wasn't until we learned about schizophrenia that we understood how to truly help him."

David's family transformation—from a source of inadvertent stress to a cornerstone of his recovery—demonstrates both the challenges and the tremendous potential of family involvement in mental health treatment. Research consistently shows that family support is one of the strongest predictors of positive outcomes for people with mental illness.[1]

THE RIPPLE EFFECT OF MENTAL ILLNESS

Mental illness doesn't occur in isolation—it affects entire family systems, creating ripple effects felt by spouses, children, parents, siblings, and even extended family members. Understanding these impacts is crucial for developing effective support strategies.

When Marcus was diagnosed with bipolar disorder, his entire family had to adjust to new realities. His sister Emma learned to recognize early warning signs of mood episodes. His parents grappled with questions about genetic risk and family history. His girlfriend had to understand that Marcus's occasional emotional intensity wasn't about their relationship but about a medical condition requiring ongoing management.

"Bipolar disorder became a family affair," Emma reflected. "It wasn't just Marcus's diagnosis—it affected how we all communicated, planned family events, and supported each other. We had to learn new ways of being together that took his condition into account."

THE BURDEN AND THE OPPORTUNITY

Family members often experience what researchers call "caregiver burden"—the physical, emotional, and financial stress associated with supporting a loved one with mental illness. Studies show that family caregivers experience higher rates of depression, anxiety, and health problems compared to the general population.[2]

Mandi's parents struggled with their own emotional reactions when their daughter's OCD began consuming hours of her day. They wondered if their parenting had contributed to her perfectionism, experienced guilt about possibly "causing" her difficulties, and felt helpless watching her struggle with rituals they couldn't understand.

"We felt like we were walking on eggshells," Mandi's mother recalled. "We wanted to be supportive, but we didn't know if giving advice would be helpful or if we should just listen. We worried that anything we said might make things worse."

However, this same closeness that creates vulnerability also creates opportunity. Families who learn about mental health conditions and develop appropriate support skills become powerful allies in recovery. They can provide emotional support, practical assistance, early warning systems for relapse, and motivation for treatment adherence.

THE SCIENCE OF FAMILY SUPPORT

Research on family involvement in mental health treatment shows consistently positive results across different conditions and populations. Studies demonstrate that family support:[3]

Reduces relapse rates by 20-40% for major mental illnesses
Improves medication adherence and treatment engagement
Decreases hospitalization rates and crisis interventions
Enhances overall quality of life for both patients and family members
Speeds recovery and improves long-term outcomes

Family support acts like a protective factor that buffers against the stresses and challenges of mental illness. Families who are educated about mental health conditions and know how to provide appropriate support essentially become part of the treatment team.

WHAT FAMILIES NEED TO KNOW: EDUCATION AS FOUNDATION

The first step toward effective family support is education about mental health conditions. Families need to understand the biological basis of mental illness, the symptoms and course of specific conditions, available treatments, and their role in the recovery process.

When Sarah was struggling with depression, her family initially tried to help by encouraging her to "just think positive" or suggesting she "count her blessings." While well-intentioned, these responses actually increased Sarah's distress because they implied that her depression was voluntary and controllable.

"Learning that depression has biological underpinnings changed everything," Sarah's sister explained. "I stopped trying to talk Sarah out of her symptoms and started learning how to support her through them. I learned when to encourage her to use her coping skills and when to just be present with her distress."

Family Education Programs

Many mental health centers now offer family education programs that provide comprehensive information about mental health conditions and effective support strategies.[4] These programs typically cover:

Understanding the Condition
Biological basis and neurochemistry
Symptoms and diagnostic criteria
Course and prognosis with treatment
Risk factors and triggers

Treatment Information
Available treatment options
How medications work and potential side effects
Different types of therapy and their goals
The importance of treatment adherence

Communication Skills
How to talk about mental health without stigma
Active listening techniques
Expressing concern without criticism
Setting appropriate boundaries

Crisis Management
Warning signs of relapse or crisis
When and how to seek emergency help
Safety planning and risk assessment
Available crisis resources

Self-Care for Family Members
Managing caregiver stress and burden
Maintaining your own mental health
Building support networks
Balancing support with enabling

"Family education transformed our relationship with David's illness," his father reflected. "Instead of feeling helpless and confused, we became knowledgeable advocates who could contribute meaningfully to his recovery."

COMMUNICATION: THE FOUNDATION OF SUPPORT

Effective family support starts with healthy communication patterns. Families dealing with mental illness often need to learn new ways of talking to each other that promote healing rather than inadvertently creating additional stress.

HIGH EXPRESSED EMOTION VS. LOW EXPRESSED EMOTION

Research has identified communication patterns that either help or hinder recovery. "High Expressed Emotion" environments—characterized by criticism, hostility, and emotional over-involvement—are associated with higher relapse rates and poorer outcomes. "Low Expressed Emotion" environments—characterized by warmth, understanding, and appropriate boundaries—promote recovery and stability.[5]

Sarah's family initially struggled with high expressed emotion patterns. When she was depressed, family members would offer constant advice, express frustration when she didn't follow suggestions, and become overly involved in trying to "fix" her mood. These responses, while motivated by love, actually increased Sarah's feelings of guilt and inadequacy.

"We learned to separate Sarah from her depression," her sister explained. "Instead of saying 'You should exercise more' or 'You need to think positively,' we learned to say things like 'I know you're struggling right now' and 'What kind of support would be most helpful?'"

Effective Communication Strategies

Families learn specific communication techniques that support recovery:

Validation: Acknowledging that the person's experiences and feelings are real and understandable, even when symptoms are involved.

"I" Statements: Expressing concerns and feelings without blame or criticism. "I worry when you don't take your medication" rather than "You're being irresponsible."

Active Listening: Focusing completely on understanding the person's perspective without immediately offering solutions or advice.

Problem-Solving Together: Collaborating to find solutions rather than imposing fixes from the outside.

Celebrating Progress: Recognizing and acknowledging small improvements and steps forward.

SETTING BOUNDARIES: LOVE WITHOUT ENABLING

One of the most challenging aspects of family support is learning the difference between helpful support and enabling behaviors that may actually impede recovery. Families need to provide love and assistance while still maintaining appropriate expectations and boundaries.[6]

Marcus's family had to learn this balance during his bipolar treatment. During manic episodes, Marcus would make impulsive financial decisions or unrealistic commitments. His family learned to provide emotional support without rescuing him from all consequences of his choices.

"We helped Marcus understand that we loved him unconditionally but that we couldn't protect him from all the consequences of decisions made during mood episodes," Emma explained. "We would help him clean up the aftermath, but we also expected him to take responsibility for his treatment and learn from his experiences."

This balance is particularly important with substance use disorders, where family members may inadvertently enable continued use by providing money, covering up consequences, or making excuses for the person's behavior.

CRISIS MANAGEMENT AND SAFETY PLANNING

Families need to know how to recognize and respond to mental health crises. This includes understanding warning signs of relapse, knowing when to seek emergency help, and having concrete plans for managing dangerous situations.[7]

Rachel's family developed a detailed crisis plan during her BPD treatment that included:

Early warning signs of emotional crisis

Specific people to contact for support
Coping strategies that had worked in the past
When to go to the emergency room
How to remove potential means of self-harm
Follow-up plans after crisis resolution

"Having a crisis plan made everyone feel more secure," Rachel's sister noted. "We weren't fumbling around trying to figure out what to do—we had specific steps to follow that had been developed when everyone was thinking clearly."

SUPPORTING TREATMENT ADHERENCE

Family members play a crucial role in supporting consistent engagement with treatment. This includes understanding the importance of medication adherence, therapy attendance, and lifestyle modifications that support mental health.[8]

David's parents learned about the importance of antipsychotic medication for preventing psychotic episodes. They helped David organize his medications, reminded him about appointments, and learned to recognize early signs that might indicate medication adjustments were needed.

"We didn't become David's medication police," his mother clarified. "But we did learn how to supportively encourage treatment adherence and how to have conversations about the importance of medication without being controlling or judgmental."

THE EXTENDED SUPPORT NETWORK

Effective support often extends beyond immediate family to include friends, colleagues, religious communities, and peer support groups. Building these broader networks provides additional resources and reduces the burden on any single family member.

Sarah's recovery was supported not just by her family, but by close friends who learned about depression, colleagues who understood her need for flexibility during treatment, and a support group where she connected with others facing similar challenges.

"Mental health recovery works best with a team approach," Sarah observed. "Different people in my network provided different types of support—emotional, practical, social, and recreational. No single person had to carry the entire burden."

PEER SUPPORT: LEARNING FROM OTHERS

Families often benefit tremendously from connecting with other families who have faced similar challenges. Peer support groups provide practical advice, emotional validation, and hope from people who truly understand the experience.[9]

David's family found great comfort in joining a family support group for people affected by schizophrenia through the National Alliance on Mental Illness (NAMI). Through these connections, they learned practical strategies, found emotional support during difficult times, and gained perspective on their own journey.

"Meeting other families who had been through similar experiences was incredibly helpful," David's father recalled. "We learned that we weren't alone, that other families had successfully navigated these challenges, and that there was reason for hope even during the most difficult periods."

CHILDREN AND MENTAL ILLNESS IN THE FAMILY

When mental illness affects a family member, children require special consideration and support. Children may not understand what's happening, may blame themselves for the family stress, or may be at increased risk for developing mental health problems themselves.[10]

Age-appropriate education helps children understand that mental illness is a medical condition, not something they caused or can cure. Children benefit from:

Simple, honest explanations about the mental health condition
Reassurance that they are not to blame
Consistent routines and support during family crises
Access to counseling or support groups designed for children
Education about their own mental health and warning signs to watch for

"We made sure our younger children understood that their sister's depression was an illness, like diabetes or asthma," one family member explained. "We told them it wasn't their fault, it wasn't something they could fix, but that there were doctors helping her get better."

CULTURAL CONSIDERATIONS IN FAMILY SUPPORT

Cultural background significantly influences how families understand and respond to mental illness. Effective support takes into account cultural values, beliefs about mental health, communication styles, and family structures.[11]

Some cultures emphasize family honor and may view mental illness as bringing shame to the family. Others have strong beliefs about the role of spirituality in healing. Some cultures have hierarchical family structures that affect decision-making about treatment

TECHNOLOGY AND MODERN FAMILY SUPPORT

Technology has created new opportunities for family support and connection. Families can now:[12]

Access online education resources about mental health conditions
Participate in virtual support groups and family therapy sessions

Use apps to track symptoms and medication adherence together
Stay connected during treatment or hospitalization
Access crisis resources and emergency services more easily

"Technology has made it easier for families to stay informed and connected throughout the treatment process," noted Dr. Chen. "Virtual family sessions allow everyone to participate even when geographic distance or scheduling conflicts would otherwise make involvement difficult."

WHEN FAMILIES STRUGGLE: PROFESSIONAL HELP FOR FAMILIES

Sometimes families need their own professional support to develop healthy ways of coping with mental illness. Family therapy can help address:[13]

Communication problems that developed during mental health crises
Caregiver burden and burnout
Guilt, blame, and relationship conflicts
Difficulty setting appropriate boundaries
The mental health needs of other family members

"Family therapy isn't just for 'dysfunctional' families," a family therapist clarified. "It's for any family that wants to learn more effective ways of supporting their loved one while maintaining their own wellbeing."

THE RIPPLE EFFECTS OF EFFECTIVE SUPPORT

When families learn to provide effective support, the benefits extend far beyond the person with mental illness. Family relationships become stronger, communication improves, and everyone develops greater resilience and coping skills.

"Dealing with David's schizophrenia was the hardest thing our family has ever faced," his father reflected. "But it also brought us closer together and taught us skills for supporting each other through any kind of crisis. We're a stronger family because of what we've been through together."

SUPPORTING RECOVERY, NOT DEPENDENCE

Effective family support aims to promote independence and recovery rather than creating dependence. The goal is to provide enough support to prevent crises while encouraging the person to develop their own coping skills and take responsibility for their treatment.

"We learned that we could love Marcus unconditionally while still expecting him to take responsibility for managing his bipolar disorder," Emma explained. "Our support helped him develop confidence in his ability to handle challenges rather than rescuing him from every difficulty."

LONG-TERM PERSPECTIVE: FAMILIES AS PROTECTIVE FACTORS

Research shows that strong family support serves as a protective factor throughout the course of mental illness. Families who maintain supportive relationships over time see:[14]

Lower rates of relapse and hospitalization
Better medication adherence and treatment engagement
Improved quality of life for everyone involved
Greater resilience during setbacks and challenges
More successful achievement of personal goals and milestones

A MESSAGE FOR FAMILIES

If your family is dealing with mental illness, remember that you didn't cause the condition, you can't cure it, but you can make a profound difference in your loved one's recovery. Your support, understanding, and advocacy can literally save lives and restore hope.

Families are often the secret ingredient in successful mental health treatment. When families are educated, supportive, and engaged, recovery rates improve dramatically. You have more power to help than you might realize.

The key is learning how to channel your love and concern into effective support strategies. This means educating yourself about mental health conditions, developing healthy communication patterns, setting appropriate boundaries, and taking care of your own mental health needs.

Recovery is rarely a solo journey. Behind every success story is usually a network of people who refused to give up, who learned how to help effectively, and who provided hope during the darkest moments. Families and support systems don't just witness recovery—they make it possible.

FOOTNOTES

1. Falloon, I. R., Boyd, J. L., McGill, C. W., et al. (1985). Family management in the prevention of morbidity of schizophrenia: clinical outcome of a two-year longitudinal study. *Archives of General Psychiatry, 42*(9), 887-896. ↩

2. Magaña, S. M., Ramírez García, J. I., Hernández, M. G., & Cortez, R. (2007). Psychological distress among Latino family caregivers of adults with schizophrenia: the roles of burden and stigma. *Psychiatric Services, 58*(3), 378-384.

3. Pitschel-Walz, G., Leucht, S., Bäuml, J., Kissling, W., & Engel, R. R. (2001). The effect of family interventions on relapse and rehospitalization in schizophrenia: a meta-analysis. *Schizophrenia Bulletin, 27*(1), 73-92.

4. Dixon, L., Lucksted, A., Medoff, D. R., et al. (2011). Outcomes of a randomized study of a peer-taught family-to-family education program for mental illness. *Psychiatric Services, 62*(6), 591-597.

5. Butzlaff, R. L., & Hooley, J. M. (1998). Expressed emotion and psychiatric relapse: a meta-analysis. *Archives of General Psychiatry, 55*(6), 547-552.

6. Meyers, R. J., & Wolfe, B. L. (2004). *Get Your Loved One Sober: Alternatives to Nagging, Pleading, and Threatening*. Center City, MN: Hazelden.

7. Stanley, B., & Brown, G. K. (2012). Safety planning intervention: a brief intervention to mitigate suicide risk. *Cognitive and Behavioral Practice, 19*(2), 256-264.

8. Velligan, D. I., Weiden, P. J., Sajatovic, M., et al. (2009). The expert consensus guideline series: adherence problems in patients with serious and persistent mental illness. *Journal of Clinical Psychiatry, 70*(Suppl 4), 1-46.

9. Solomon, P. (2004). Peer support/peer provided services underlying processes, benefits, and critical ingredients. *Psychiatric Rehabilitation Journal, 27*(4), 392-401.

10. Beardslee, W. R., Versage, E. M., & Gladstone, T. R. (1998). Children of affectively ill parents: a review of the past 10 years. *Journal of the American Academy of Child & Adolescent Psychiatry, 37*(11), 1134-1141. ↩

11. Alegría, M., Atkins, M., Farmer, E., Slaton, E., & Stelk, W. (2010). One size does not fit all: taking diversity, culture and context seriously. *Administration and Policy in Mental Health and Mental Health Services Research, 37*(1-2), 48-60. ↩

12. Glynn, S. M., Cohen, A. N., Murray-Swank, A. B., et al. (2006). A family intervention with relapse prevention training for schizophrenia. *American Journal of Psychiatry, 163*(12), 2156-2158. ↩

13. McFarlane, W. R., Dixon, L., Lukens, E., & Lucksted, A. (2003). Family psychoeducation and schizophrenia: a review of the literature. *Journal of Marital and Family Therapy, 29*(2), 223-245. ↩

14. Hooley, J. M. (2007). Expressed emotion and relapse of psychopathology. *Annual Review of Clinical Psychology, 3*, 329-352. ↩

CHAPTER 11
LIVING WITH MENTAL ILLNESS – A MESSAGE OF HOPE

Recovery does not look the way we often imagine it should.

When someone receives a diagnosis of serious mental illness—schizophrenia, bipolar disorder, major depression, schizoaffective disorder, obsessive-compulsive disorder, or borderline personality disorder—the initial hope is usually for a return to baseline. Get treatment. Take medication. Do therapy. Get better. Return to normal life.

For many people, this narrative of recovery must be revised. Not because recovery is impossible—it absolutely is possible—but because recovery often means something different than "going back to how things were." Recovery, in the lived experience of people managing serious mental illness, means achieving functional improvement, building a meaningful life within the context of ongoing symptoms, and reclaiming dignity and purpose despite ongoing challenges.

This chapter tells the story of six individuals we've met throughout this book—Sarah, Marcus, James, David, Mandi, and Rachel—each living successfully with mental illness years into their treatment journeys. Their stories share common themes: the critical importance of biological interventions, the power of consistent daily management strategies, the transformative impact of addressing stigma and building genuine community, and the quiet, profound hope that comes from learning to live well rather than chasing the fantasy of complete cure.

Sarah's Return: Depression and the Long Road to Stability

Sarah, the marketing manager, is now in her tenth year of stable treatment, advanced to director of marketing, and has rebuilt her relationship with her daughter. Her stability rests on combination medications—an SSRI antidepressant plus a low-dose mood stabilizer plus an anti-anxiety medication—combined with cognitive-behavioral therapy that taught her to recognize and manage depressive thought patterns.[1] She maintains consistent sleep, exercises regularly, and recognizes her early warning signs of depression. "I'm not cured," Sarah said. "I'll always need medication. But I'm functional, present with my daughter, successful at work. That's recovery for me."

Marcus: Bipolar Disorder and the Freedom of Stability

Marcus, the software engineer, is now 33 and five years into stable treatment with lithium. He leads a team of engineers, has a committed relationship, and remains acutely aware that his stability rests on consistent biological intervention. "Lithium is not glamorous, but it's the most effective medication I've ever taken for preventing mood episodes," Marcus noted. "Research shows people with bipolar disorder who stay on lithium have dramatically lower rates of suicide and hospitalization."[2] He maintains the lifestyle habits he learned in treatment: consistent sleep, regular exercise, stress management, and immediate action when symptoms emerge. "The medication isn't limiting me—it's enabling me to be the person I want to be."

James: Schizoaffective Disorder and the Power of Combination Treatment

James, the architect, has been in treatment for seven years and works part-time freelancing on architectural projects. His stability rests on combination medications: an antipsychotic (paliperidone via monthly injection), a mood stabilizer (valproic acid), and an antidepressant (sertraline). "I'm on three medications because my illness is complex and requires a multifaceted approach," James explained. "The antipsychotic addresses the voices and paranoid thoughts. The mood stabilizer helps prevent mood cycling. The antidepressant manages depressive episodes."[3] Beyond medication, he maintains a structured daily routine, engages with a therapist and peer support group, and works with his partner to recognize early warning signs of symptom worsening. "Without the antipsychotic, I cannot think clearly or work or maintain relationships. With it, I can build a life," James said.

David: Schizophrenia and Redefining Success

David is now 25, six years into treatment for schizophrenia. He lives in a supervised apartment, volunteers at an animal shelter, and has found community through a peer support group. His antipsychotic medication (via monthly injection) has reduced his hallucinations and paranoid thoughts, though negative symptoms—lack of motivation and emotional flatness—remain his greatest challenge. "I'm not going back to engineering school," David said matter-of-factly. "That part of my life is over. But I've learned to find meaning in what I can do. Working with animals gives my day structure and purpose."[4] Early diagnosis and consistent treatment may have prevented a more severe trajectory. "Medication is not optional for us," David emphasized. "It's the foundation."[5]

Mandi: OCD and the Role of Targeted Intervention

Mandi, with OCD, represents a different trajectory of recovery where specific targeted interventions are essential. High-dose SSRI medication (100mg daily) forms her foundation, but the medication alone was insufficient without cognitive-behavioral therapy specifically adapted for OCD called exposure and response prevention (ERP).[6] "The medication alone didn't help my OCD. I needed therapy where I intentionally expose myself to my obsessive thoughts and resist compulsions," Mandi explained. Years into treatment, she continues her SSRI, practices ERP techniques, and maintains lifestyle habits that support her recovery. "I used to spend hours a day on compulsions. Now I might spend twenty minutes a day. That's a massive improvement in functioning and quality of life."

Rachel: Borderline Personality Disorder and Dialectical Behavior Therapy

Rachel, age 26, has spent the past four years in dialectical behavior therapy (DBT), a comprehensive treatment program specifically designed for borderline personality disorder. She now works as a peer counselor, directly supporting others with serious mental illness. Unlike psychotic or mood disorders, Rachel's recovery has been built primarily on behavioral and psychotherapeutic intervention rather than medication.[7] "DBT is intense—individual therapy, group skills training, phone coaching—but it's worth it," Rachel explained. DBT taught her emotion regulation, distress tolerance, interpersonal effectiveness, and mindfulness skills. "I used to hurt myself regularly when emotions became overwhelming. Now I have other options," she said. Her recovery demonstrates that while biological interventions are foundational for many illnesses, psychological and behavioral interventions can be equally transformative for others.

The Foundation: Biological Interventions Across the Spectrum

One theme emerges unmistakably from the stories of these six individuals: biological interventions form the foundation upon which recovery is built.

For Sarah with depression, the combination of SSRI and mood stabilizer creates the neurochemical stability required to do therapy work and maintain functional behavior. For Marcus with bipolar disorder, lithium prevents the devastating cycles of mania and depression that otherwise recur. For James with schizoaffective disorder, the combination of antipsychotic, mood stabilizer, and antidepressant addresses the multifaceted neurological dysfunction underlying his illness. For David with schizophrenia, the antipsychotic medication reduces hallucinations and delusions enough to make functional living possible. For Mandi with OCD, the high-dose SSRI reduces the intrusive nature of obsessive thoughts enough to allow behavioral therapy to work. And for Rachel with borderline personality disorder, psychiatric medications managed her acute symptoms while intensive behavioral therapy became her primary tool for recovery.

The emphasis on biological interventions reflects a fundamental truth: serious mental illness arises from brain dysfunction. While psychological interventions, lifestyle modifications, and social support are all essential, they work optimally when the biological substrate is treated. A person in psychosis cannot benefit from therapy until antipsychotic medication reduces the severity of hallucinations and delusions. A person in severe depression cannot implement behavioral changes without the medication that provides enough neurochemical stability to take action. A person with OCD cannot tolerate exposure therapy without the SSRI medication that reduces anxiety enough to make the therapy tolerable.

This is not to diminish the importance of other interventions. All of our six individuals combine medication with therapy, lifestyle management, and social support. But the biological intervention—the medication—is foundational.[8] Without it, recovery, as these individuals have achieved it, would not be possible.

Daily Strategies: Living Well with Mental Illness

Beyond medication, all six individuals practice consistent daily strategies that support their stability. These strategies are not glamorous or revolutionary—they are the unglamorous, consistent fundamentals of mental health management.

Sleep hygiene is universal. All six prioritize consistent sleep schedules, adequate sleep duration, and sleep quality. They recognize that sleep disruption destabilizes mood and exacerbates psychotic and obsessive symptoms. Marcus jokes, "Sleep is better than any medication I take. If I'm getting seven to eight hours consistently, everything feels more manageable."

Routine and structure create containers that support stability. David relies heavily on structure—consistent times for waking, medication, meals, volunteer work, and evening routines. Without structure, his motivation (already compromised by negative symptoms) evaporates entirely. Mandi uses structured exposure exercises as part of her OCD management. Sarah maintains consistent work hours and exercise times, knowing that unstructured time increases her vulnerability to depressive thoughts.

Exercise is nearly universal in our six individuals' lives. They exercise not because they enjoy it (though some do) but because they understand intuitively or through therapy that exercise powerfully affects mood and anxiety. Marcus swears by running as his primary stress management tool. David finds structure and purpose in his volunteer work but also engages in regular walks. Sarah does both resistance training and aerobic exercise, finding that the combination helps both her mood and her sleep.

Stress management and boundary-setting are essential. James practices meditation. Marcus uses mindfulness. Rachel uses dialectical behavior therapy skills. Sarah has learned to say no to work commitments that would overwhelm her. All six have learned to recognize their personal warning signs of symptom worsening and to respond proactively—contacting their psychiatrist, intensifying therapy, and prioritizing self-care before symptoms escalate.

Social connection and support are essential, though they look different for each individual. Sarah has rebuilt relationships and recently married. Marcus is open about his bipolar disorder with close friends. James has a partner and therapy support. David has found community in a peer support group. Mandi has close relationships and works in mental health supporting others. Rachel works as a peer counselor and has built meaningful friendships. None of them are living in isolation. All have recognized that recovery requires connection.

Addressing Stigma and Building Community

Perhaps the most powerful aspect of recovery, as these six individuals experience it, is the transformation that comes from addressing stigma and building genuine community.

For years, all six internalized the stigma surrounding their illnesses. They saw themselves as broken, damaged, lesser-than. They hid their diagnoses, felt shame about needing treatment, and believed that their mental illness defined their entire identity and value.

Recovery has meant, in part, dismantling that internalized stigma.

"I used to introduce myself mentally as 'Sarah with depression,'" Sarah reflected. "My depression was the first thing I thought about when I woke up. Now, yes, I still take antidepressants and work on my mental health. But that's not my identity. I'm a marketing director, a mother, a partner, a person who happens to manage depression. That shift changed my entire self-concept."

Marcus is explicit about his bipolar disorder with people close to him. "If I'm going to ask my team to shift deadlines because I need to prioritize my mental health, or if I'm going to need accommodations at work, I have to be honest about why. And when I'm honest, people are usually much more understanding than I expected."

James advocates for better understanding of schizoaffective disorder, writing articles and speaking to groups. "Stigma thrives in silence and ignorance," he said. "When I talk openly about my condition, I reduce both. And I model for other people with mental illness that you can be open and still be respected and valued."

David and Rachel both participate in peer support and advocacy. David speaks to family groups about early signs of schizophrenia. Rachel works as a peer counselor, directly supporting others with serious mental illness. Both have found that their lived experience, far from being a liability, is their greatest strength in helping others.

Mandi has become vocal about OCD in her community, pushing back against the popular cultural trivialization of the disorder. "People joke about being 'so OCD' when they mean they like things organized," she said. "Real OCD is debilitating. By being open about my experience, I help people understand what it actually is."

All six have benefited from community—whether through therapy support, peer support groups, professional networks, or families that have learned about their conditions. All recognize that hiding their mental illness increases suffering, while openness, combined with appropriate boundaries, creates connection and support.

Recovery, in this sense, is not about hiding mental illness or pretending to be "normal." It's about integrating mental illness into one's identity while refusing to allow it to define one's entire sense of self-worth or possibility.

Redefining Recovery as Functional Improvement

Perhaps the most important shift in understanding these six individuals' lives is the redefinition of recovery itself.

If recovery means "return to pre-illness baseline with no symptoms," then most of these individuals have not recovered. Sarah still takes multiple psychiatric medications daily. Marcus will likely need lithium indefinitely. James manages persistent psychotic symptoms despite medication. David continues to hear voices and struggle with motivation. Mandi still has obsessive thoughts and compulsive urges. Rachel still struggles with emotional regulation.

But if recovery means "achieving functional improvement, building a meaningful life within the context of ongoing symptoms, reclaiming agency and dignity, and finding purpose despite ongoing challenges," then all six have clearly recovered.[9]

Sarah works as a director. She has rebuilt her relationship with her daughter. She has a committed partnership. She engages in regular exercise and meaningful activities. She manages her symptoms and her life successfully. This is recovery.

Marcus leads a team of engineers. He has built a stable, loving relationship. He advocates for mental health. He manages his symptoms and his life successfully. This is recovery.

James works in his field, maintains a partnership, builds meaningful relationships, and manages his symptoms and his life. This is recovery.

David lives independently with support, volunteers meaningfully, has built community, and finds purpose. This is recovery.

Mandi works in mental health supporting others, has meaningful relationships, and manages her symptoms. This is recovery.

Rachel works as a peer counselor, helps others, has meaningful relationships, and has built a stable life. This is recovery.

None of their recoveries look like what they initially imagined. But all of them, by any meaningful measure, represent genuine recovery and functional improvement.

The Message of Hope

What should people newly diagnosed with serious mental illness take from these stories?

First, treatment works. This cannot be overstated. Medications, therapy, lifestyle interventions, and support all work. The evidence is overwhelming: people with depression, bipolar disorder, schizophrenia, OCD, schizoaffective disorder, and borderline personality disorder can achieve significant improvement with appropriate treatment.[10]

Second, recovery is achievable, though it may look different from what you initially imagined. You may not return to your pre-illness baseline. You may continue to experience symptoms. You may need ongoing treatment. But you can build a functional, meaningful life. You can work, maintain relationships, contribute to your community, and experience satisfaction and purpose.

Third, biological interventions, such as medications, TMS and sometimes ECT are essential for most serious mental illnesses. This is not weakness. This is not giving up. This is engaging with the biological reality of brain dysfunction and using our most powerful tools to address it. Taking medication is an act of self-care and wisdom, not a sign of failure or abnormality.

Fourth, medication works best when combined with other interventions: therapy, lifestyle modifications, social support, and meaningful activity. Recovery is multifaceted and requires attention to the biological, psychological, social, and existential dimensions of mental health.

Fifth, addressing stigma—both external and internalized—is crucial for recovery. Hiding mental illness increases suffering. Being open, within appropriate boundaries, creates connection and reduces shame. Your mental illness is a part of you, but it is not all of you.

Sixth, recovery is not linear or guaranteed. There will be setbacks. There will be periods of symptom worsening. You may need medication adjustments or therapy modifications. But with persistence and appropriate support, recovery is possible.

Finally, you are not alone. Millions of people manage serious mental illness. Many of them, like Sarah, Marcus, James, David, Mandi, and Rachel, are building functional, meaningful lives. Their stories prove that mental illness, while serious and sometimes devastating, is not a life sentence to dysfunction and despair. It is a manageable medical condition that, with appropriate treatment and support, can be integrated into a life that is rich, purposeful, and worth living.

A FINAL WORD

I have had the privilege of working with thousands of individuals navigating mental illness over three decades of psychiatric practice. I have witnessed the transformative power of accurate diagnosis, evidence-based treatment, and compassionate support. I have seen lives rebuilt, relationships restored, and purpose reclaimed.

But I have also witnessed something equally important: I have watched people like Sarah, Marcus, James, David, Mandi, and Rachel transform not only their own relationship with mental illness but also the relationships of those around them. By being open about their struggles, by engaging fully in treatment, by building meaningful lives, and by speaking truth about their experiences, they have changed how their families, friends, colleagues, and communities understand mental illness.

This is the deeper message of hope. Mental illness, far from being shameful or hopeless, can become, paradoxically, a source of profound learning and growth. Not because mental illness is good—it is not. It is serious, sometimes devastating, and deeply challenging. But in the struggle to reclaim life despite mental illness, many individuals discover resilience, compassion, connection, and purpose they might never have found otherwise.

If you or someone you love is navigating mental illness, I hope these stories offer not false hope but genuine, evidence-based hope: the hope that treatment works, that recovery is possible, that functional improvement is achievable, and that a life of meaning and purpose awaits you.

This hope is grounded in science, clinical experience, and the lived experience of millions of individuals managing serious mental illness successfully. It is the hope that has sustained me through my career and that I offer to you now.

You are not broken. You are not hopeless. You are managing a treatable medical condition. With proper treatment, appropriate support, and persistence, recovery is possible. Not recovery as a fantasy of returning to how things were, but recovery as a lived reality of building a life that is functional, meaningful, and worth living.

That is what I wish for you.

FOOTNOTES FOR CHAPTER 11

1. Ruberto, A., Zaki, N., Tamás, V., & Arolt, V. (2014). Combination therapy in major depressive disorder: A narrative perspective. *Therapeutic Advances in Psychopharmacology*, 4(4), 174-184.

2. Cipriani, A., Hawton, K., Stockton, S., & Geddes, J. R. (2013). Lithium in the prevention of suicide in mood disorders: updated systematic review and meta-analysis. *BMJ*, 346, f3646.

3. Bauer, M. S., Wisniewski, S. R., Marangell, L. B., et al. (2006). Predictors of response to treatment in first-episode bipolar disorder in the Systematic Treatment Enhancement Program for Bipolar Disorder (STEP-BD). *Journal of Affective Disorders*, 94(1-3), 51-58.

4. Lieberman, J. A., Drake, R. E., Sederer, L. I., et al. (2008). Science and recovery in schizophrenia. *Psychiatric Services*, 59(5), 487-496.

5. Marshall, M., Lewis, S., Lockwood, A., Drake, R., Jones, P., & Croudace, T. (2005). Association between duration of untreated psychosis and outcome in cohorts of first-episode patients. *Archives of General Psychiatry*, 62(9), 975-983.

6. Abramowitz, J. S., Franklin, M. E., & Foa, E. B. (2011). Empirical status of cognitive-behavioral therapy for obsessive-compulsive disorder: a meta-analysis. *Romanian Journal of Cognitive and Behavioral Psychotherapy*, 1(1), 1-26.

7. Linehan, M. M., Comtois, K. A., Murray, A. M., et al. (2006). Two-year randomized controlled trial and follow-up of dialectical behavior therapy vs therapy by experts for suicidal behaviors and borderline personality disorder. *Archives of General Psychiatry*, 63(7), 757-766.

8. Kamenov, K., Cabello, M., Caballero, F. F., et al. (2017). The relationship between health and life satisfaction: A mediation analysis. *Quality of Life Research*, 26(12), 3371-3383.

9. Walker, E., Shapiro, D., Esterberg, M., & Trotman, H. (2010). Neurodevelopmental origins of psychosis in the offspring of affected parents. *Biological Psychiatry*, 57(10), 1057-1066.

10. Rounsaville, B. J., Carroll, K. M., & Onken, L. S. (2001). A stage model of behavioral therapies research: Getting started and moving toward more advanced stages. *Clinical Psychology: Science and Practice*, 8(2), 133-142.

APPENDIX: MENTAL HEALTH RESOURCES

CRISIS SUPPORT & EMERGENCY RESOURCES

National Suicide Prevention Lifeline

Phone: 988 (call or text) **Available:** 24/7 **Website:** suicidepreventionlifeline.org Crisis counselors provide free, confidential support to anyone in suicidal crisis or emotional distress. Call or text 988 to connect with a trained counselor.

Crisis Text Line

Text: HOME to 741741 **Available:** 24/7 **Website:** crisistextline.org Text-based crisis support for those who prefer to reach out via text message.

National Domestic Violence Hotline

Phone: 1-800-799-7233 (1-800-799-SAFE) **TTY:** 1-800-787-3224 **Text:** START to 88788 **Available:** 24/7 Support for victims of domestic violence and those concerned about a loved one.

SAMHSA National Helpline

Phone: 1-800-662-4357 **Available:** 24/7, free and confidential **Website:** samhsa.gov Referrals to local mental health and substance use treatment facilities, support groups, and community-based organizations.

Veterans Crisis Line
Phone: 988, then press 1 **Text:** 838255 **Chat:** veteranscrisisline.net **Available:** 24/7 Specialized support for veterans and their loved ones in crisis.

MENTAL HEALTH ORGANIZATIONS & SUPPORT

National Alliance on Mental Illness (NAMI)
Phone: 1-800-950-NAMI (6264) **Website:** nami.org **Helpline:** Monday–Friday, 10 a.m.–10 p.m. ET NAMI provides education, advocacy, and peer-to-peer support for individuals and families affected by mental illness. Resources include support groups, educational programs, and community events. NAMI also offers specialized support for specific conditions including depression, bipolar disorder, schizophrenia, and anxiety disorders.

NAMI Resources:
Local affiliate chapters throughout the US
Support groups and educational classes
Peer-run programs and peer specialists
Family support and education programs
Advocacy and stigma-reduction initiatives
Mental health screening tools
Multilingual resources

Mental Health America (MHA)
Phone: 1-800-969-6642 **Website:** mhanational.org Provides screening tools, resource directories, and educational information about mental health conditions and treatments.

Depression and Bipolar Support Alliance (DBSA)
Phone: 1-800-826-3632 **Website:** dbsalliance.org Peer-led support groups and educational programs specifically for depression and bipolar disorder.

Anxiety and Depression Association of America (ADAA)
Phone: 1-240-485-1001 **Website:** adaa.org Educational resources, support, and therapist finder for anxiety and depression.

The National Association of Social Workers (NASW)
Website: helpstartshere.org Find licensed clinical social workers and mental health resources by zip code.

TREATMENT & PROVIDER RESOURCES

Brainsway, Inc. – TMS Treatment Provider Locator
Website: brainsway.com **Provider Locator:** brainsway.com/find-a-center **Zip Code Search:** Available on their provider locator Brainsway specializes in Transcranial Magnetic Stimulation (TMS) therapy, an FDA-approved, non-invasive treatment for depression and other mental health conditions. Use their zip code locator to find TMS treatment centers near you. Contact centers directly to inquire about specific conditions treated and insurance coverage.

SAMHSA Treatment Locator
Website: findtreatment.samhsa.gov **Phone:** 1-800-662-4357 Comprehensive directory of mental health and substance use treatment facilities, with filters by location, insurance, and specialty services.

Psychology Today Therapist Finder
Website: psychologytoday.com Search for licensed therapists and psychiatrists by zip code, insurance, and specialty.

TherapyDen
Website: therapyden.com Online therapist directory with filtering by location, insurance, and treatment specialty.

Betterhelp & Talkspace
Websites: betterhelp.com / talkspace.com Online therapy platforms offering virtual sessions with licensed therapists (availability of platforms varies by state).

Substance Abuse and Mental Health Services Administration (SAMHSA)
Website: samhsa.gov Federal agency providing information about mental health and substance use treatment, prevention, and recovery support.

SPECIFIC CONDITION RESOURCES

Schizophrenia & Psychotic Disorders
National Alliance on Mental Illness (NAMI): nami.org/schizophrenia
Schizophrenia and Related Disorders Alliance of America: sardaa.org
Early Psychosis Intervention Network: epi-network.org

Bipolar Disorder
Depression and Bipolar Support Alliance: dbsalliance.org **International Bipolar Foundation:** ibpf.org **Bipolar 1 Support:** bipolar1support.org

Anxiety Disorders
Anxiety and Depression Association of America: adaa.org **National Institute of Mental Health – Anxiety:** nimh.nih.gov/anxiety

Depression
National Institute of Mental Health: nimh.nih.gov/depression **Depression and Bipolar Support Alliance:** dbsalliance.org **American Foundation for Suicide Prevention:** afsp.org

Borderline Personality Disorder
National Education Alliance for Borderline Personality Disorder: neabpd.org **DBT Self Help:** dbtselfhelp.com

ADHD
CHADD (Children and Adults with ADHD): chadd.org **Phone:** 1-800-233-4050

PTSD & Trauma
National Center for PTSD: ptsd.va.gov **International Society for the Study of Trauma and Dissociation:** isst-d.org

PEER SUPPORT & SUPPORT GROUPS

Depression and Bipolar Support Alliance (DBSA)
Website: dbsalliance.org In-person and online peer support groups led by individuals with lived experience.

NAMI Connection Recovery Support Groups
Website: nami.org/support-groups Free, peer-led support groups for people in recovery from mental health conditions.

AA, NA, and Related 12-Step Programs
Alcoholics Anonymous: aa.org / 1-212-647-1680 **Narcotics Anonymous:** na.org / 1-888-6-NANA-WEB **Adult Children of Alcoholics:** adultchildren.org

Online Support Communities
7 Cups: 7cups.com (free emotional support chat) **Mental Health Reddit Communities:** reddit.com/r/mentalhealth, r/depression, r/bipolar, etc.

EDUCATIONAL RESOURCES & BOOKS

Foundational Books on Mental Health Recovery

- *The Body Keeps the Score* by Bessel van der Kolk – Trauma and recovery
- *Emotional Intelligence* by Daniel Goleman – Understanding emotions and emotional regulation
- *Man's Search for Meaning* by Viktor Frankl – Finding purpose in adversity
- *The Myth of Sanity* by Marya Hornbacher – Mental illness narratives and recovery
- *An Unquiet Mind* by Kay Redfield Jamison – Bipolar disorder memoir
- *The Bell Jar* by Sylvia Plath – Depression and mental health fiction
- *Darkness Visible* by William Styron – Depression memoir
- *Feeling Good* by David D. Burns – Cognitive behavioral therapy approaches

Books on Specific Treatments

- *DBT Skills Training Manual* by Marsha Linehan – Dialectical Behavior Therapy
- *Cognitive Therapy and the Emotional Disorders* by Albert Ellis – Cognitive Behavioral Therapy foundations
- *The Bipolar Workbook* by Monica Ramirez Basco – Practical tools for bipolar management

Memoirs & Personal Stories

- *Turtles All the Way Down* by John Green – Anxiety and OCD
- *Girl, Interrupted* by Susanna Kaysen – Mental health hospitalization
- *My Anxious Mind* by Mark S. Goulston – Anxiety management

GOVERNMENT & RESEARCH RESOURCES

National Institute of Mental Health (NIMH)

Website: nimh.nih.gov **Phone:** 1-866-615-6464 Federal research institute with evidence-based information on mental health conditions, treatments, and clinical trials.

National Institutes of Health (NIH)

Website: nih.gov Research and clinical trial information across all areas of health and mental health.

Substance Abuse and Mental Health Services Administration (SAMHSA)

Website: samhsa.gov Federal agency supporting prevention, treatment, and recovery services for mental health and substance use disorders.

FDA – Mental Health Drug Information

Website: fda.gov Information about FDA-approved medications and treatments for mental health conditions.

ClinicalTrials.gov

Website: clinicaltrials.gov Search for ongoing clinical trials for mental health treatments and conditions.

WORKPLACE & DISABILITY RESOURCES

Equal Employment Opportunity Commission (EEOC)
Website: eeoc.gov Information about workplace rights and protections under the Americans with Disabilities Act (ADA).

Job Accommodation Network (JAN)
Website: askjan.org **Phone:** 1-800-526-7234 Free consultation on workplace accommodations for employees with disabilities, including mental health conditions.

Employee Assistance Programs (EAP)
Check with your employer's HR department for available EAP services, which typically provide free confidential counseling and referral services.

CRISIS PREVENTION & SAFETY PLANNING

Create a Safety Plan
Work with a mental health professional to develop a personalized safety plan that includes:

Warning signs that a crisis may be developing
Internal coping strategies you can use on your own
People and social settings that provide distraction
People you can ask for help
Professional contacts and crisis lines
Means restriction (reducing access to means of self-harm)

International Association for Suicide Prevention

Website: iasp.info/resources/Crisis_Centres/ International crisis center directory.

ADDITIONAL SUPPORT RESOURCES

Family Support

National Alliance on Mental Illness (NAMI) Family Support: nami.org Educational programs and support groups specifically for families and loved ones.

Caregiver Resources

Caregiver Action Network: caregiveraction.org Support and resources for those caring for individuals with mental health conditions.

LGBTQ+ Mental Health

Trevor Project: 1-866-488-7386 / thetrevorproject.org **LGBTQ+ National Youth Talkline:** 1-800-246-7743

Racial & Ethnic Minority Mental Health

National Alliance on Mental Illness (NAMI) Communities of Color: nami.org **Therapy for Black Girls:** therapyforblackgirls.com **National Suicide Prevention Lifeline (Spanish):** 1-888-628-9454

Veterans Resources

Veterans Affairs Mental Health: mentalhealth.va.gov **Veterans Crisis Line:** 988, then press 1

HOW TO USE THESE RESOURCES

If you're in immediate crisis: Call 988 (Suicide & Crisis Lifeline) or go to your nearest emergency room.

If you're seeking treatment: Start with SAMHSA's National Helpline (1-800-662-4357) or use the SAMHSA Treatment Locator (findtreatment.samhsa.gov) to find facilities near you.

If you're looking for support groups: Contact NAMI (1-800-950-NAMI) or DBSA (1-800-826-3632) to find peer-led groups in your area.

If you're supporting someone else: Call NAMI's helpline to speak with someone who can guide you through the process of supporting a loved one.

If you're struggling with stigma: Reach out to NAMI's advocacy programs or mental health organizations focused on your specific condition.

A FINAL WORD

These resources represent a starting point in your journey toward mental health and recovery. Whether you're seeking help for yourself or supporting a loved one, remember that reaching out is a sign of strength, not weakness. The mental health community is filled with compassionate professionals and peer supporters who are ready to help.

Your mental health matters. Your recovery is possible. Help is available.

www.ingramcontent.com/pod-product-compliance
Lightning Source LLC
LaVergne TN
LVHW050933210926
848482LV00013B/601
* 9 7 9 8 9 9 3 7 7 9 4 0 9 *